Praise for
HIDDEN MEDICINE

"As a psychiatrist who has studied spirituality's role in health for decades, I find the clinical-theological vision of *Hidden Medicine* a much-needed practical complement to the extensive empirically grounded research, offering hope to those for whom conventional medicine has fallen short.

Dr. McCormack's bold, groundbreaking book challenges the status quo and illuminates a path toward wholeness that few have dared to chart. He shows that healthcare without attention to the spirit is incomplete—and that true healing is possible when spirituality is embraced. A must-read for anyone seeking holistic transformation."

—Harold G. Koenig, MD, MHSc, Professor of Psychiatry and Behavioral Sciences and Associate Professor of Medicine, Duke University School of Medicine; author, *The Healing Power of Faith: How Belief and Prayer Can Help You Triumph Over Disease*

"*Hidden Medicine* is not just a book—it's a battlefield map. Dr. McCormack courageously pulls back the veil on a war that most of modern medicine refuses to acknowledge.

As someone who overcame a terminal brain cancer diagnosis by confronting the unseen forces that traditional medicine ignores, I found the concept of Ruachiatry both revolutionary and deeply resonant. Dr. McCormack's stories, from spiritual encounters to clinical breakthroughs, reveal the profound truth that healing must go beyond the physical.

This is a must-read for anyone seeking true wholeness—body, mind, and spirit. It will challenge your worldview, deepen your faith, and offer hope where the system has failed. I'm grateful this book exists."

—Dr. Pete Sulack, founder, Redeem Health & Chiropractic and Matthew 10 International; author, *Be Resilient* and *The Joseph Blessing*

"This is a book we've needed for a long time—one born of hard-won insight, both in the clinic and in the crucible of spiritual warfare. Dr. McCormack and I underwent a challenging season of spiritual opposition, and I witnessed firsthand his perseverance through the attacks. It was in the wake of that experience that he and I first discussed coauthoring a book on this very subject. After several brainstorming meetings, I told him what had become clear: This was his book to write.

Drawing on his extensive medical experience and profound spiritual understanding, Dr. McCormack writes with wisdom and authority—the right voice at just the right time in which there is so much uncertainty in the world. I urge you to read *Hidden Medicine* now and to read it to the very end. It is a rare book that carries the potential to bring deep healing, lasting peace, and clarity for those who find themselves in the unseen battles of life."

—David Mills, PhD, Senior Pastor, Beallwood
Baptist Church; former Professor of Evangelism,
Southwestern Baptist Theological Seminary

"Dr. Thomas McCormack dares to raise issues I've never heard a fellow psychiatrist discuss in my nearly forty years in the field, much less a triple-boarded, Duke-trained child and adolescent, adult, and forensic psychiatrist.

In *Hidden Medicine*, Dr. McCormack presents a compelling argument that the biopsychosocial model that shapes our understanding of medical and mental illness often fails us because it fails to account for spiritual forces that influence health and well-being. One may agree or disagree with his arguments, but Dr. McCormack's writing will cause patients and clinicians alike to consider other explanations for illness, disease, and suffering."

—Stephen Grcevich, MD, founder and president, Key Ministry;
author, *Mental Health and the Church: A Ministry Handbook for Including
Children and Adults with ADHD, Anxiety, Mood Disorders,
and Other Common Mental Health Conditions*

"As a traditionally trained medical doctor who has transitioned into functional medicine, I look at all aspects of my patients in a very holistic manner. An individual is more than just a body, and their mind, emotions, and spiritual state play an essential role in their overall health and happiness.

Dr. McCormack's book is an excellent text that focuses on an area of every person's life that unfortunately most medical professionals overlook today. I strongly suggest that any medical practitioner who really cares about the needs of their patients, as well as anyone who is concerned about their overall well-being, read this book and put into practice the important principles that Dr. McCormack lays out. It is a greatly needed and valuable resource."

—Paul C. Broun, MD, physician and
former US Congressman from Georgia

"I've known Dr. McCormack for more than fifty years. He is a rare person possessing both broad scientific knowledge and an unshakeable faith—and *Hidden Medicine* brilliantly bridges both worlds. I promise that you have never read anything like this.

This unique book has the potential to transform how physicians care for patients in mind, body, and spirit. Its powerful prescription for patients still struggling with physical and mental illnesses despite standard medical treatments is nothing short of revolutionary."

—Russell Biven, WVLT Channel 8 broadcaster;
former television news anchor, WBIR
Channel 10; former sports anchor, CNN

"As a pastor who has spent countless hours counseling people, I could not be more grateful for this work by Dr. McCormack. *Hidden Medicine* is a refreshing approach to helping people that accounts for the whole person—body, mind, and spirit. It also directly addresses the often overlooked yet essential aspect of the spiritual realm in the diagnostic and healing process.

I have read numerous books on counseling, but I have never read anything that has more potential for true transformation than this. *Hidden Medicine* will not only be an indispensable resource for professional and pastoral counselors, but it will also be a great help to anyone to reads it. I recommend it unreservedly and with great enthusiasm."

—J. Josh Smith, DMin, Senior Pastor, Prince Avenue Baptist Church; author, *The Titus Ten: Foundations for Godly Manhood*

"Dr. McCormack is a man of deep Christian faith whose authenticity shines forth in this helpful volume in which he makes the case that faith and spirituality are the very basis of health and life itself. This book is pastoral and compassionate yet scholarly and reasonable. Above all, it is based on eternal truth that will refresh some readers and uncover new pathways to healthy thinking and living for others. To all it will affirm our position as people of worth who are offered wholeness in life when we align our will with that of the Great Physician.

As a pastor of almost sixty years, I highly recommend this long-awaited book for the troubled, the caregivers, and the seekers of truth and lasting wholeness. Dr. McCormack helps us understand things that may cause many of our struggles in life but without being sensationalistic or overly simplistic. You will gain insight into a new path to health in addition to those that involve pills, syringes, or surgeries. A must-read!"

—Stewart D. Simms, Jr., MDiv, DMin, Pastor Emeritus, Beech Haven Baptist Church; author, *Words Not Spoken: Understanding the Pastor's Silent Hurts*

"As a Licensed Clinical Pastoral Counselor, I meet with individuals and families who love God and love each other yet are suffering. They are suffering through difficult relationships, painful memories, and childhood trauma, among other things. In all of these conversations, I address the truth that they are created in the image of God with spirit, soul, and body. Very often, the client has never considered nor understood this truth and how it impacts their healing and wholeness. In *Hidden Medicine*, Dr. McCormack provides both client and counselor explanation, insight, and guidance on how to incorporate these spiritual truths into their healing journey.

I have known Dr. McCormack for nearly twenty years through professional and personal avenues. His reputation in our community is one of personal integrity, sound wisdom, strong faith, and professional expertise. His book meets an important need in the counseling community."

—Windy Echols, MA, NCCA Licensed Clinical Pastoral
Counselor, Encompass Christian Counseling

HIDDEN MEDICINE

HIDDEN MEDICINE

The UNSEEN WAR *on Your* HEALTH *and the*
SPIRITUAL PRESCRIPTION *for* HEALING
that COULD TRANSFORM HEALTHCARE

THOMAS McCORMACK, MD

GREENLEAF
BOOK GROUP PRESS

Published by Greenleaf Book Group Press
Austin, Texas
www.gbgpress.com

Copyright © 2025 Thomas Wayne McCormack, Jr.

All rights reserved.

Thank you for purchasing an authorized edition of this book and for complying with copyright law. No part of this book may be reproduced, stored in a retrieval system, used for training artificial intelligence technologies or systems, or transmitted by any means, electronic, mechanical, photocopying, recording, or otherwise, without written permission from the copyright holder.

Distributed by Greenleaf Book Group

For ordering information or special discounts for bulk purchases, please contact Greenleaf Book Group at PO Box 91869, Austin, TX 78709, 512.891.6100.

Design and composition by Greenleaf Book Group
Cover design by Greenleaf Book Group
Cover images used under license from ©Adobestock.com
For permissions credits, please see page 340, which is a continuation of the copyright page.

Publisher's Cataloging-in-Publication data is available.

Print ISBN: 979-8-88645-411-6

eBook ISBN: 979-8-88645-412-3

To offset the number of trees consumed in the printing of our books, Greenleaf donates a portion of the proceeds from each printing to the Arbor Day Foundation. Greenleaf Book Group has replaced over 50,000 trees since 2007.

Printed in the United States of America on acid-free paper

25 26 27 28 29 30 31 32   10 9 8 7 6 5 4 3 2 1

First Edition

To my patients, whose courage and stories have deepened my understanding of healing, and to all who seek wholeness in body, soul, and spirit—may this book illuminate your path and guide you toward the hidden truths that bring true healing.

CONTENTS

Prologue

DO YOU WANT
TO BE HEALED?

Picture yourself at the doctor's office—my office. You have come to seek help for a severe emotional disorder that has not responded to standard medical and psychological treatments. This disorder is having a significant negative impact on your life, and your physician has referred you to me because I have extensive experience dealing with "treatment-resistant" cases like yours.

Although you were reluctant to see a psychiatrist, you researched my credentials and seem satisfied that my requisite education, training, and more than twenty-eight years of experience practicing medicine at least qualify me to possibly help you. But, I'm a little different—I delve into the spiritual contributions to illness, an area with which most physicians are uncomfortable. I had extensive religious education for six years while attending a Roman Catholic college preparatory school. I then received my undergraduate education at Wake Forest University, where I graduated with honors with a bachelor's degree in history. Afterward, I achieved my life-long dream of becoming a physician when I earned my medical degree from Emory University. The next six years of my formal education and training were at Duke University, where I completed a residency in general psychiatry, a fellowship in child and adolescent psychiatry, and a second fellowship in forensic psychiatry. I earned board certification status in all three specialties and have been a clinical professor at two medical schools—Emory and currently at the University of Georgia. Additionally, after many years of being a skeptical agnostic, I am now a person of faith who has been ordained as a deacon at a local congregation.

After taking a history, performing many tests, and conducting a thorough evaluation of your medical and emotional problems, I question you about your spiritual life.

You respond: "I guess you'd say I'm fairly spiritual. I believe in God, but I try not to go to extremes or be judgmental. I attend worship services when I can, but I don't think God has a problem if I sleep in occasionally. I do pray sometimes, mostly when I really need help, but I'm not great at making it a daily habit because I am really busy. I know I should read scripture more, but I just don't have the time. I do believe scripture is generally true, but I don't think it's realistic to follow every single thing it says. I believe we have a soul that lives on after we die, but I'm not sure what the afterlife looks like. I try not to think too much about it and just be in the moment in this life. I'm not sure I really believe in hell—I think that may be something religions made up to scare their followers into compliance. I just have a hard time believing that a good and loving God would send anybody to a place of eternal fire and torment. I try hard to treat others the way I would want to be treated. I guess I'm basically a good person, so whatever is next, I'm confident I'll be okay."

The results of your tests, your history, and your examination confirm to me what I suspected—you are indeed quite sick. In fact, you have two very serious illnesses and continue to suffer because a large component of each has been completely overlooked, leading you to receive the wrong treatments.

"The first diagnosis is that you are blind, spiritually speaking. Unbeknownst to you, the charismatic and powerful leader of unseen spiritual forces has blinded your mind since birth.[1] He has done so because he is by nature a liar, who uses deception to confuse and mislead you, making it difficult for you to recognize the truth and accept the facts that will lead you to the only cure available for your other malady.[2] But there is a self-existent higher spiritual power who created all other lesser spiritual entities, including your powerful, deceptive enemy. The good news is this all-powerful Spirit is both willing and able to open the eyes of blind people like you.[3]"

I hesitate momentarily before continuing: "I regret to inform you of even more troubling news—you have a terminal illness."[4]

Solemnly I continue, "I know this is not what you were expecting to hear and that your first and perfectly normal response will likely be denial. But the truth is that you must accept this dire reality before we can discuss any treatment. In fact, along the way, there will be other difficult-to-accept truths with which you will have to grapple. So, I have one question for you before I discuss the next steps in your treatment. Do you want to be healed?"

What? you think to yourself. You feel like flippantly answering such a seemingly obvious question with "Of course—that's why I'm here!" But instead, you simply nod, overwhelmed by the alarming diagnoses I have just given you.

"The good news is there is a cure," I continue. "The bad news is I don't have it. While most well-intentioned doctors offer treatments to help their patients' underlying symptoms or numb their pain, only one physician in the entire world offers the cure. I happen to know this physician well, and I can refer you to him if you are interested. But first, I must warn you that he is controversial; while some say he has the power to perform miraculous healings, others say he is crazy, and yet others say he is a fraud and a huckster.

"But because this doctor is independently wealthy, cares deeply for people who are suffering, and genuinely wants to see no one die, he graciously offers the cure for free![5] I have known this physician personally for more than thirty-two years now, and I can tell you that I wholeheartedly believe him to have the ability to heal when traditional means have failed. I once heard of a man whom he healed who had been paralyzed from the waist down for thirty-eight years. When traditional medicine had offered him no help, this desperate man sought a miraculous healing by turning to superstitions that were unsupported by scientific evidence. Despite the paralytic's misguided faith, a serendipitous meeting with this physician led to him being fully healed after only one brief visit, in which he was asked the very same question—do you want to be healed?"[6]

Although you are skeptical, you agree to see this physician because of the gravity of your situation. *What do I have to lose?* you ponder.

"I am very pleased you have bravely decided to be open-minded, setting aside your preconceptions regarding what steps it takes to achieve a cure," I continue. "This is the place where most people stop their journey and decide to passively continue down the comparatively easier broad road and take the mainstream medical treatments that are not curative but work by either numbing the senses or distracting patients from their suffering."

Still struggling to come to terms with all of this, you inquire, "Why doesn't everybody who has my illness see this doctor who has the cure? And why have I never heard of it?"

I explain that one reason is that access to the truth about this healer and the cure he offers is hidden by mankind's unseen spiritual enemies, who influence the people who control the currently widely available treatments. "The battle you and others face to obtain this free cure is not against the powerful health insurance companies, the pharmaceutical industry, or their lobbyists," I say. "In fact, your battle is not against flesh-and-blood human beings at all but rather spiritual principalities and powers who hate God and by extension hate you for being the object of his affection, created in his own image.[7]

"You heard me correctly. Just as you believe in the existence of atoms or the wind, even though you have never seen either one, you must grasp the reality that spiritual beings, whom you have also never seen, do indeed exist and are actively involved in the running of our physical world. Most major religious faiths of the world acknowledge the existence of such spiritual enemies.

"The reason you have never heard of this absolutely free cure is that those running the show put up great resistance to being exposed. They have become accustomed to their status, positions of prominence, wealth, influence, power, and to being almost deified for their creativity and supposed intellectual genius. They are more than willing to fight to maintain this status and will use any means at their disposal, especially censorship of information, misinformation, or even outright lies. One of their tactics is to accuse their detractors of the exact same morally bankrupt activities in which they are involved. They get away with it because they are a part of the machine, a worldwide system run by powerful enemies who operate from behind the scenes. This machine consists of multiple powerful arms to provide them backup, such as government, the healthcare industry, big business, the educational system, and law enforcement.

"But there is one thing I ask you to do before I refer you to the doctor holding the cure," I say as I hand you a book. "This is a book I've written titled *Hidden Medicine*. It is essential that you read it before seeing this doctor, because it will give you valuable insight into spiritual realities and the ongoing opposition to your healing, along with a brief overview of the treatment for your terminal condition. I know this is scary, and there is much uncertainty, but I have learned how to fight these malevolent forces because I share the same terminal illness, and as a physician, I have helped thousands of others who have it over the years. As you read my book, be humble, open-minded, willing to accept certain uncomfortable facts, doggedly determined, and a sincere seeker of truth. We'll meet again once you have finished it."

I rise and walk you to the door, shaking your hand before you exit. "Goodbye for now," I say, "and remember—there is always hope. You just need to know where to find it."

Section I

SPIRITUAL REALITIES

1

UNSEEN FORCES

To my own shock, the last years in the western world have opened me up for the first time to the belief that there may be a devil . . . It is almost impossible to explain the rejection of what is good and the celebration of what is wrong so radically and so quickly without recourse.

—DENNIS PRAGER, "BIBLICAL SERIES: EXODUS" PODCAST SERIES, *THE DAILY WIRE*

*C*rash!

It was just after 10 p.m. in our rental home in Granada, Nicaragua. I was peacefully nestled in bed, reading. My wife was asleep next to me. Our three young kids were in bedrooms across the small courtyard from ours. Suddenly, something shattered outside the window. I was startled and immediately leaped up. Cautiously, I ventured outside to investigate.

When we'd arrived earlier that day, at our upscale rental in the middle of the city, we'd all gotten some creepy vibes. The high-fenced walls surrounding the small compound were topped with barbed wire, and eerie photos and paintings of a little child adorned the walls throughout the premises. When we asked about them later, we were told by the rental agency that the son of the woman who owned the place had tragically died at a young age. She desired to preserve his memory by hanging macabre paintings and photos of him throughout her home.

"Kids!" I bellowed as I entered the courtyard.

Immediately, three terrified little faces peered out from their bedroom windows. A large concrete planter situated right outside their bedrooms had fallen and crashed to the ground, collapsing into a pile of soil and flowers in the courtyard. The night was still. There was no wind or adverse weather of any kind, and yet, somehow, this very substantial urn had fallen. My three children were understandably frightened, but after I comforted them and explained that a flowerpot had accidentally tipped over, they calmed down and went back to their beds. I slipped back into bed myself and began reading again.

Fifteen minutes later, I heard something land on the tin roof above our bedroom, followed by footsteps. It sounded like a large animal. Then the clawing began. For five minutes straight, I listened to something pouncing on the tin roof, followed by high-pitched scratching sounds. Then I heard what sounded like dozens of clenched fists simultaneously banging on the roof. My heart and mind raced. My first thought was that it was some kind of dangerous pack of wild animals. My second thought was that perhaps it was criminals who had broken in to terrorize us.

My wife woke up and was immediately frightened. This was very unusual for her. I began praying aloud, and after several minutes, I ended the prayer with, "In the name of Jesus Christ, I command you to leave now!" Immediately, there was a loud thunderclap, and all the commotion stopped. Still petrified, I grabbed the walking stick in the corner of the room and stepped outside.

There was nothing there. Nothing.

I turned on all the lights and backed up a distance to examine the roof. Nothing.

I checked on the kids. They'd heard it all and were terrified. But I could give them no explanation.

All five of us slept in the same crowded bed that night.

We were not bothered the rest of the week.

To this day, I have no scientific rationale for what we experienced that frightening night in Nicaragua.

The Rise of Unexplained Phenomena

When I was a child growing up in the 1970s and '80s, strange phenomena like this were a rare, spooky novelty. While most of the stories were easily explained by natural phenomena or debunked as hoaxes, there remained a few unexplained cases presented by seemingly high-functioning, intelligent, reliable witnesses who had no motive for lying. Occasionally, these rare cases ended up on a television show, such as *In Search of . . .* or *Unsolved Mysteries.*

I recall being fascinated by these phenomena, wondering if they were objectively real or the product of one's vivid imagination—or perhaps even a mental illness. But because these phenomena were so rare, people generally dismissed them and even ridiculed the witnesses as crackpots.

The day after Christmas 1973, the film *The Exorcist* was released, capturing the imagination of audiences the world over. The screen adaptation of William Peter Blatty's 1971 novel was said to be loosely based on an actual case: the demonic possession of a boy in Baltimore that occurred after he and his aunt played with a Ouija board. No story like that had ever been told on the big screen.

Unlike the world before 1973, accounts of these phenomena are much more common today. They are prevalent in the mainstream media, and paranormal shows are now a staple of primetime television and streaming networks, like the History Channel and the

Travel Channel. Movies claiming to be about real-life paranormal events like those in *The Exorcist* are popular and quite lucrative. *The Conjuring* movie series, about famed demonologists Ed and Lorraine Warren, is one of many examples.

The curious might wonder what the reason is for the marked increase in these strange phenomena and the public's insatiable appetite for recounting such terrifying tales. Is it just mass delusion? Mankind's primal fear of things that go bump in the night? Or perhaps it's just imagination run amok from our fear of harm or death at the hands of some evil force outside our control?

In sensational, purportedly supernatural cases, we certainly need to first rule out psychological phenomena, substance intoxication, and mental or physical illness as the cause. I've spent more than two decades doing this very work with thousands of patients. Often, such causes are the culprits. But when these causes are clinically ruled out, I believe the only remaining answer is the fact that there exists an invisible, spiritual realm, whose inhabitants seem increasingly willing to step out from behind the shadows. Given the rapid, unsettling changes in the world today, many people—like Mr. Prager—are more open to this possibility. If this unseen realm does indeed exist, then the most reasonable source for further investigation into this theory would be the world's major religious traditions.

The Spiritual Roots of Illness

These religions all describe evil spiritual enemies of mankind. They're called *Asuras* in both Hinduism and Buddhism, *Shedim* in Judaism, *jinn* in Islam, and *demons* in Christianity. Hindus also believe in other malevolent spirits they call *Rakshasas* (demonic beings) and *Pishachas* (flesh-eating spirits) that harm humans, cause chaos, and oppose divine order. Adherents to these religious faiths believe that these unseen enemies have been waging an invisible war against us for many centuries, especially against religious leaders. For example, the Buddha was believed to have been tempted during his enlightenment by an evil, Asura-like figure called Mara. Similarly, following his baptism, Jesus was tempted by an evil spiritual being called Satan during a forty-day fast in the wilderness.

According to the world's three major monotheistic religions, there is a single, all-powerful God, who at a specific time in the distant past created all things, and his creation was good. There were both spiritual created beings, collectively called *elohim* in the Jewish Tanakh, which includes our modern conceptualization of angels, and corporeal created beings called *mankind*. Each lived in their own realm, and the two realms initially overlapped. Judaism teaches of such a spiritual realm populated by angelic *Malachim* and malevolent *Shedim*. Similarly, Islam teaches that Allah created spiritual beings from "smokeless fire,"[1] who are called *jinn* and are capable of good or evil.

According to the Judeo-Christian worldview, the realities of our experience—like sickness, physical decline, death, separation of the physical and spiritual realms, and a cosmic war between rebellious spiritual beings and humans—were not part of God's original plan for creation, including for mankind. These were the consequences of rebellion against God. The Bible states that God himself will return and re-create the Edenic environment he originally intended and that redeemed mankind will live forever in bodies free from sin and corruption. Until then, mankind has been relegated to life in a fallen physical realm of which sickness is a large part. The past 300 years have seen incredible advancements in our understanding of these physical and mental maladies, yet many people still receive insufficient or only temporary relief from traditional medical treatments.

When Medicine Fails Against the Enemy of Illness

As a physician, I have seen many instances in which sickness either does not have the typical presentation or does not follow the typical course of a known disease or disorder. Some of these unusual cases also do not respond to normally effective, well-established medical treatments. How do we explain these cases, when scientific rationale evades us after we have conducted a thorough history, physical examination, and laboratory and imaging studies? Often, doctors do not know what to make of these puzzling cases. As a last resort, they refer them to a psychiatrist, like me.

I have come to view illness, both physical and mental, as an enemy that we need to fight. We often hear about a patient's "battle with cancer" or about "the war on drugs" fought by the millions afflicted with addiction. These phrases are more accurate than we might realize.

The modern method of combating most common physical illnesses is to employ highly educated and trained physicians, such as internists, pediatricians, and family physicians, who are on the front lines of the battle. For more rare maladies or those requiring very detailed knowledge and technical skill, we have an army of subspecialists to call upon when needed. Additionally, there are psychiatrists and other mental health professionals available to help with maladies of the *psyche*, the Greek word for "soul"—that is, the mind, emotions, and the will.

But what if the weapons we healthcare providers employ are inadequate to help patients in their fight? Is it possible that we are missing a key component to our understanding and treatment of illness?

The Missing Spiritual Component

My opinion is that the answers to these questions lie in the belief that mankind is a tripartite being, composed of body, soul, and spirit. In the field of medicine, clinicians are trained to apply the biopsychosocial model proposed by George Engel in 1977 to the diagnosis and treatment of both physical and mental illness.[2] This approach takes into account many factors related to the presentation and cause of illness: physiological pathology, genetic vulnerabilities, temperament, IQ, cognitions, emotions, behaviors, coping methods, personality structure, education, interpersonal relationships, and economic, environmental, and cultural influences. However, this abundance of considerations addresses only the body and soul of a patient. It overlooks the spiritual element in the individual's life.

The idea that true healing requires an integration of body, mind, and spirit is not new. It's deeply rooted in the wisdom of ancient religious traditions. Hinduism, for instance, views the human being as a complex interplay of the physical (*sthula*), subtle (*sukshma*), and causal (*karana*) bodies, all of which must be aligned for health and harmony. Similarly, Jewish mysticism, through the lens of Kabbalah, teaches that disruptions in spiritual balance can manifest as physical illness, emphasizing the need for deeper spiritual healing.

In Islamic tradition, maintaining spiritual health is seen as essential to overall well-being. The concept of *jihad al-nafs*—the internal struggle against one's lower desires—parallels the idea that unresolved spiritual conflicts can impact both mental and physical health. Buddhism teaches that liberation from suffering requires the cultivation of awareness and the dissolution of ignorance (*avidya*).

We have millions of doctors trained to diagnose and treat maladies of both the body and the soul. But what about diagnosing and treating maladies occurring in the realm of an individual's spirit? Who are the practitioners tasked with healing spiritual sickness or combating spiritual contributions to physical and mental illnesses?

Many people erroneously think that pastors, priests, rabbis, and imams carry this mantle, but most often these individuals are called by God to shepherd his people and preach and teach the religious truths of their faith. While there is often some degree of pastoral counseling involved in their theological education, this is not a primary area of focus for most religious leaders. Today, there is very little overt acknowledgment of demonic influence in peoples' maladies, outside of deliverance ministries, which are most common in Christian Pentecostal circles, and the rare rite of exorcism performed by a priest ordained to do so by the Roman Catholic Church. Offered even less is a direct spiritual intervention other than prayer or brief pastoral counseling.

This puzzles me, especially since multiple sacred texts clearly provide evidence that some medical, neurological, and psychiatric problems are directly due to the influence of demons. Regardless of whether one believes Jesus of Nazareth to be the Son of God, he is esteemed by billions of believers and skeptics alike for his extraordinary wisdom concerning the human condition.[3] His views of the spiritual realm are front and center in the many ancient documents that record him performing miraculous healings of physical ailments caused by demonic spiritual forces. Examples from the Bible include kyphosis (humpback),[4] epileptic seizures,[5] convulsions and foaming at the mouth,[6] mutism,[7] and severe mental illnesses that prompted aggression and self-harm.[8]

This spiritual component of healing, a significant factor in Jesus's well-documented life, is most often relegated to the less scientifically rigorous fields of alternative and complementary medicine. Practitioners in these fields are very often pagan (as defined by the *Oxford English Dictionary*: "a person holding religious beliefs other than those of the main world religions"). Unfortunately, this leaves adherents to the world's major religions—more than three-quarters of the global population[9]—without help for spiritual maladies from a practitioner who holds the same beliefs they do. What would this mean if a significant percentage of the world's maladies had a spiritual component?

Goals of This Book

I have two main goals in writing this book.

First, I hope to awaken you to the realities of the spiritual realm, equipping you to fight and win these unseen battles with malevolent forces.

My second goal applies to the medical community in particular. It is my opinion that physicians and other healthcare providers must be taught and trained to incorporate spiritual realities into their medical practices. I believe this is more straightforward than it seems. While the world's five major religions—Judaism, Christianity, Islam, Buddhism, and Hinduism—differ in significant ways, they still share many of the same spiritual principles, beginning with the belief that the spiritual realm exists and is essential to one's health.

This addition of the spiritual component to the well-established treatments of body and soul is what I term *Ruachiatry* [Roo-uh-ky-uh-tree], derived from the Hebrew word *ruach* [Roo-aak], meaning "spirit." Because of the inherent challenges in integrating the spiritual with established biological and psychological subject matter, I have sought expert guidance from several respected theologians and pastors.

All this being said, I have no desire to impose my beliefs on my readers or my patients. As a physician, I view as sacred the autonomy and free will of patients to make their own decisions about their healthcare, without any undue influence from a practitioner. It is my duty to inform patients of my opinions regarding their maladies and possible treatment options. Armed with knowledge from a caring, educated, and experienced physician, it is the patient's job alone to weigh the information, accept or reject it, and make subsequent decisions. I ask the same of you as you read this book.

As I will explain, my spiritual belief system came from an initial stance of intellectual skepticism. However, I had an encounter with a supernatural being that convinced me there was indeed a God. I felt a strong sense of responsibility to discover who he was and what religious system best led to knowledge of and a relationship with him. I strongly encourage you to also embrace this responsibility and decide for yourself what you believe, then eventually become fully capable, as I am now, of giving a coherent, rational defense for the beliefs that you hold. I believe with all my heart that the humble, open-minded seeker of truth will indeed find it. And finding answers to the fundamental questions of our origins, who we are, and what our unique purpose is in life is worth the effort. As Socrates famously asserted, "The unexamined life is not worth living."[10]

The universality of these ideas—found in sacred texts, spiritual practices, and cultural healing traditions—points to a shared human understanding: that health is more than the absence of disease. It's a state of balance between body, mind, and spirit. Whether it's the Jewish practice of *Cheshbon HaNefesh* (soul accounting), the Buddhist pursuit of enlightenment through mindfulness, the Hindu alignment of energy centers (*chakras*), or the Islamic call to purify the heart (*tazkiyah al-nafs*), traditions across the world recognize the need for deeper, holistic healing.

Considering Spiritual Causes

When the natural order of things is overridden to bring about something good, believers call it a miracle and attribute it to a benevolent higher power. So, when the natural order of things is overridden to bring about wickedness, should we not consider that spiritual enemies could be behind it? When negative circumstances in our own lives, especially regarding our health, are unusual, extraordinary, or altogether defy a rational, natural explanation, they at least warrant deeper examination. In these cases, after all other potential causes have been ruled out, I believe we should ask the question: Is it possible that malevolent, invisible enemies could be behind this? And, if so, what can we do about it?

In the pages to come, I will attempt to answer these questions, both as an experienced physician who desires to lead my patients to wholeness and as an individual who desires wholeness for myself and those I love.

2

WHAT YOU DON'T KNOW CAN HURT YOU

If I were the devil . . . I'd set about however necessary to take over the United States. I'd subvert the churches first—I'd begin with a campaign of whispers. With the wisdom of a serpent, I would whisper to you as I whispered to Eve: "Do as you please." . . . If I were the devil, I'd take from those who have, and give to those who want until I had killed the incentive of the ambitious. And what do you bet I could get whole states to promote gambling as the way to get rich? I would caution against extremes and hard work in patriotism, in moral conduct. I would convince the young that marriage is old-fashioned, that swinging is more fun, that what you see on the TV is the way to be. And thus, I could undress you in public, and I could lure you into bed with diseases for which there is no cure.

In other words, if I were the devil I'd just keep right on doing what he's doing.

—PAUL HARVEY, "IF I WERE THE DEVIL" BROADCAST

The Unseen Battle You're Already In

You may not know it, but you're in a fight.[1]

You live on a battleground, not a playground. And if you are unaware of this fact, you will likely become a casualty, easy prey for experienced enemy soldiers.

You didn't pick this fight; in fact, you might consider yourself a generally peaceful person. But you're in a fight nonetheless, and it is unjust—you don't deserve this. Unbeknownst to you, you are a pawn in a greater invisible cosmic war between an all-powerful creator God and less powerful, created spiritual beings who rebelled against his authority a long time ago. While not omnipotent, your unseen enemies are quite formidable, and they typically fight dirty.

These demonic foes have an immensely gifted and charismatic leader, whose main character trait is pride.[2] He and his minions do not follow the typical rules of engagement in battle. They have a win-at-any-cost mentality, relentlessly employing guerrilla warfare, hitting below the belt, and taking no prisoners in the process.

Your enemy's ultimate sinister goal is to steal, kill, and destroy anything that brings you life.[3] So far, the enemy has been successful at times in stealing your joy, peace, energy, focus, pleasure, and sleep, leaving you unproductive in your work, socially isolated, tired, unmotivated, and despondent. This enemy army, in some cases, kills those against whom it wages war, and its demonic soldiers relish their ability to destroy marriages, families, health, employment, and one's future.

You are beaten down and tired. You are wounded, but there is no reprieve from the battlefield, because your enemy oppresses you each and every day. Sure, some days are better than others, but you feel as though you're drowning, because you can never get your head above water for very long before you are pushed back down under. You feel alone and without hope. You feel like throwing in the towel.

I know how you feel.

My Encounter with Spiritual Warfare

Years ago, thinking I was equipped as a spiritually mature believer with a wide knowledge of Scripture and as an ordained leader of deacons at a local church, I foolishly, naively, and arrogantly picked a fight with malevolent spiritual forces. I grossly overestimated my abilities and simultaneously underestimated my unseen enemy. I lost, big time. In fact, I was absolutely routed. I can only imagine what defeat is like for those who don't even realize that an invisible war rages all around them. They are destined to become collateral damage, caught in the cross fire of this unseen but very real conflict.

During the healing and recovery that followed my own spiritual defeat, I resolved to learn all I could about my demonic foes. I discovered that it is indeed possible to endure suffering as a good soldier while undergoing training to become a warrior, not a casualty, in the cosmic invisible war.[4]

The culmination of these efforts is this book, in which my deepest desire is to impart to you the knowledge I have gained. I hope to equip you to fight and win the battles you face in your own life.

What follows does not merely derive from my own personal experience but also from my clinical experience as a psychiatrist for more than twenty-five years, evaluating and treating thousands of patients in many settings, including both public and private mental hospitals, academic centers, jails, prisons, public mental health centers, and, most recently, in private practice.

Recognizing Evil in Psychiatric Cases

My interest in soul sickness and the problem of evil in the world led me to pursue a career in psychiatry, followed by subspecialty training in forensic psychiatry. Working in a maximum-security federal prison that housed a mental hospital, I came to believe that, while socioeconomic status, education, personality traits, history of abuse or neglect, substance abuse, and biological factors all play a role in producing criminal, antisocial behavior, evil was a difficult-to-define but very real and tangible force.

When I met evil, I knew it almost instinctively. I'm not talking about people who occasionally commit a sin like the rest of us mortals. I am talking about people who seem to lack basic morals and values and easily disregard others as objects to be used or obstacles in their way. The people infected with it are not like you and me. They look right through you with a cold, menacing stare. They hate you without reason. They hurt others and seem to lack remorse. They seem almost nonhuman, as if an invisible entity to whom they submitted long ago is malevolently directing their lives. Evil is more than misdeeds; it is organized, planned, and purposeful malice.

It was during my forensic psychiatry fellowship that I began to study sociopathy and the question of evil. Where did evil come from? Was it simply the product of ingrained patterns of persistent antisocial behavior? Or was evil something separate, something that had a hidden hand behind its malevolent intentions? If there is a good God, why does he allow evil to exist in the first place?

Through my research, I discovered that God did not create evil itself, nor did he create evil beings. Contrary to popular opinion, he did not create the Devil as I once erroneously supposed. Instead, God created a beautiful, intelligent, highly gifted cherub named Lucifer, who became the Devil only when he rebelled against his Creator, according to the Jewish Tanakh.[5] According to Islamic theology, there was a jinni named Iblis, who was a devout servant of Allah until he rebelled by refusing to bow down to Adam, to whom Iblis felt he was superior. As with Satan in Judeo-Christian theology, the God of Islam then cursed this rebellious spiritual adversary and banished him from paradise, where he now attempts to lead humans astray until the coming day of judgment. This first historical record of evil shows us the clear, demonstrable template that evil does not originate in God, nor is it woven into the fabric of creation by divine decree. Evil is the perversion of God's good gift of free will—the decision to depart from God's intended path, seeking one's own ends by one's own means. This exercising of self-will above God's will is idolatry in its most subtle form and the height of arrogance, in which the perpetrator breaks the first of God's commandments by ostensibly enthroning him or herself as God.[6]

Through the course of my career as a psychiatrist, I have not only dealt with cases of evil that seemed to have an unseen force behind the sinister words and actions of its perpetrators but also clinical patients who complained of "intrusive thoughts," which were often distressing in their content and seemed foreign to them, perhaps sown by invisible interlopers. In contrast to individuals with antisocial personality disorder, these patients saw such thoughts not as their own but as what they perceived them to be—unwelcome intruders they did not know how to remove. Whereas patients with antisocial personality disorder seemed to provide a welcoming environment or even invite negative spiritual energy, these clinical patients seeking help seemed more like unwitting victims whose intruders took advantage of their neglect to hold down the fortress of their mind. Many of them seemed to have inadvertently left a door cracked open for an invader to enter.

Over my career, I have also encountered occasional cases of strange and scientifically unexplainable phenomena in reports from my clinical patients and in events I have witnessed in the clinic. Early in my career, I assumed that patients' tales of seeing ghosts or demons or hearing a sinister voice were simply psychopathology, the product of a biochemically diseased brain.

Certainly, some patients, especially those with severe persistent psychotic disorders such as schizophrenia, fit this bill. Others with personality disorders could likewise experience phenomena they misconstrued as demonic, especially in times of heightened stress. Furthermore, in the Bible Belt where I practiced, it was not uncommon for manic patients to experience religious delusions, such as beliefs they had received special messages or assignments from the spiritual realm.

But the cases that puzzled me most involved patients who were relatively high functioning, with stable interpersonal relationships, families, and job histories. They had no other symptoms of psychotic pathology but seemed to be genuinely afflicted by unseen forces construed as foreign and outside of themselves. I became determined to understand the cause of the unexplainable symptoms in my patients, and over time I began to see certain common characteristics among these cases.

Integrating Spirituality into Medical Practice

As I said earlier, seeing these patterns in many of those afflicted, I came to believe that certain "doors" could be left open, making it quite easy for spiritual intruders with ill intentions to gain access. Common open doors often included dabbling in the occult, alcohol and drug abuse, illicit and unnatural sex, pornography, and/or a history of severe trauma. Such open doors seemed to provide the unseen enemy with a toehold, which over time became a foothold, which eventually degraded into a stronghold in the patient's mind. Essentially, the enemy broke in, took control, and refused to leave, building an impregnable fortress.

The more I progressed in my own spiritual journey, the more tuned in I became to the spiritual realm. Somewhat concurrently, more patients felt comfortable divulging their experiences of the supernatural, both positive and negative. I believe this was likely due to the fact that I was somewhat of a unicorn—a trusted, non-judgmental therapist who was open to the possibility of an unseen spiritual realm and a psychiatrist who did not instantly assume all such talk was the product of delusions and hallucinations.

I began to increasingly use spiritual aspects, in addition to the biological, psychological, and social aspects I had been trained to employ, when hypothesizing the causes of my patients' complaints. I came to believe that it was vital to discern the degree to which each of these various aspects contributed to the issue that a patient was seeking to remedy.

In medicine, in order to prescribe the appropriate treatment intervention, it is paramount for the practitioner to correctly identify the underlying causes or contributing factors to the presentation of the patient's particular illness. Regrettably, the profession of medicine has long been unwilling to address potential spiritual contributions to illness. This is most likely because the profession deemed such a pursuit unscientific and more applicable to the realm of theology, and thus better left for clergy to address.

For years, I didn't know what to make of the relatively common phenomenon of otherwise high-functioning, cognitively lucid patients describing visual hallucinations of shadow people or demonic entities or auditory hallucinations of a menacing voice saying blasphemous or self-deprecating comments and/or urging the patient to hurt themselves or take their life.

Early in my career, I assumed the symptoms were the product of a mind plagued by psychosis, and so after a thorough medical workup, including a brain MRI and extensive blood tests, I often initiated treatment with an antipsychotic medication, resulting in varying degrees of success. But I have experienced rare moments in both the emergency department and the clinic over the years that have left me much more open-minded to the possibility of demonic influence in such cases.

When Science Can't Explain: Strange Clinical Encounters

During the course of my general psychiatry residency at Duke, I was taught that people under the influence of certain drugs, especially PCP (also known as "angel dust"), would not only experience psychotic symptoms but also at times exhibit superhuman strength. Back then, police body-camera footage was not generally released to the public, so I was skeptical, despite the widespread reports.

Around that time, I heard a sermon on the radio by a renowned pastor, who recounted a chilling incident his friend, a state trooper, had told him about. The suspect, who was high on PCP, came toward the trooper with a knife and refused the command to stand down. Subsequently shot with a shotgun multiple times at close range, the suspect continued to come after the officer before finally collapsing. I recall believing that the reason for this was that PCP is an anesthetic, and the suspect was simply numb and couldn't feel the pain from the gunshots. My thoughts on the subject changed a few months later when I personally encountered a patient who was high on PCP in the emergency department.

In the 1990s, the Duke University Medical Center emergency department was very busy with psychiatric patients, partly due to the prevalence of substance abuse in the area. I was told that Durham, North Carolina, was a unique spot on the East Coast, given that two interstate highways ran through the city on a major drug-running route from Washington, DC, to Miami. While on call one night, I was awakened at 2 a.m. and asked to see a drug-intoxicated patient who'd been brought in by police. By the time I arrived, the man was restrained, yelling incoherently, and thrashing about, trying to break through his restraints. I ordered an intramuscular injection of the antipsychotic haloperidol and a sedative in an attempt to calm him. It didn't work. I ended up ordering two more injections over the course of the next hour.

Normally, the large doses he was given would put a patient to sleep, but they merely calmed this man to a degree so that I could enter the padded room and converse with him. I do not recall the specifics of what he told me, only that his words were the delusional ramblings of a madman.

I spoke with the arresting officer, who stated that the patient was causing a public disturbance and that it had taken six officers and a stun gun to subdue him. Due to the danger this patient posed to others, I made the decision to admit him to the psychiatric ward for drug detoxification and treatment of his psychosis.

I'll never forget what happened next. I have rarely spoken of it.

A young nurse and I went into the room with the patient to determine if he was calm enough to be released from his restraints for transfer to the ward.

"You're going to be admitted to the hospital," I explained to the patient, "and we will go as soon as you're out of those restraints and calm."

He listened, then said, "Okay."

Since he had been relatively calm for an hour or so, the nurse and I cautiously undid his restraints.

Slowly, almost methodically, he sat up on the stretcher, and for a brief moment he looked at us as if he were sizing us up. Then he flashed a creepy grin, bolted toward the wall on the opposite side of the room, and climbed it, like Spider-Man. He paused halfway up— crouching on all fours in defiance of gravity—to look back at us.

The young nurse and I ran for the door, bursting into the hall-way, both of us calling for help. A security guard and two techs rushed in to find the man sitting on the floor smiling.

I do not mean to insinuate that this is necessarily a case of demonic involvement, but I have no rational, medical explanation for what I witnessed.

I do believe that this case highlights the notion that illicit, mind-altering substances, especially ones with hallucinogenic prop-erties, may somehow open a gateway to the spiritual realm. In my opinion, my patient's untreated schizophrenia possibly cracked the door open to the demonic realm, but the substance he ingested likely blew the door wide open, allowing the inexplicable phenom-enon to occur.[7]

A more recent example is that of a middle-aged woman who had been seeking treatment by psychotherapists and psychiatrists for many years. She had a significant history of trauma, which had largely remained unaddressed in her therapy, due to the sensitive and painful nature of it. In childhood, she had been abandoned by her father and experienced repeated sexual abuse perpetrated by her brother.

In addition to post-traumatic stress disorder, she suffered from severe and persistent depression that had not responded to mul-tiple medication trials, psychotherapy, electroconvulsive therapy, transcranial magnetic stimulation, or even implantation of a vagus nerve stimulator. Further complicating matters were her new emp-ty-nester status and difficulties in her marriage.

During one of our visits, her moods were unusually erratic. She started off angrily confronting me about why none of the treatments had seemed to be very effective and threw in some personal jabs at me for good measure. I calmly explained that she had a very difficult, refractory case and reminded her that I had referred her to another psychiatrist for a second opinion as well as a treatment-resistant depression clinic at a reputable medical school. I told her that I shared her frustration, wasn't going to give up, and would be happy to continue working with her, if she desired. When she began sobbing uncontrollably, I felt there was nothing further I could say to comfort her, so I decided to sit with her in her pain.

I began to pray for her silently as she sobbed.

Her demeanor and posture suddenly changed. She went from uncontrollably crying, with her face buried in her hands, to abruptly sitting up straight on the couch, more agitated and belligerent than before. Then she turned her head slowly in my direction. I could see that her demeanor was different, even her eyes, which stared at me intensely.

Then she spoke in a voice I'd never heard come out of her.

"Stop that! It's not going to work!" growled a deep, creepy voice that emanated from her lips. Her stare was piercing, cold, and menacing. Whatever was speaking, it did not seem to be my sweet-but-troubled patient. I immediately felt I was in the presence of something possibly supernatural and potentially evil.

I did not know how to respond, so I addressed the patient.

"Carrie"—not her real name—"what in the name of Jesus is going on?"

I had specifically invoked the name of Jesus, in case there might be a spirit involved in her sudden disturbing behavior. This tactic has been widely reported to provoke supposed evil spirits, who generally have a strong aversion to anything holy.

Immediately, my patient slithered down off the couch in a serpentine fashion onto the floor and appeared to be writhing in pain as deep guttural sounds emanated from her mouth. I moved closer to examine her and make sure she was okay. Then suddenly, she sat up and lunged at me, grabbing and breaking my glasses and scratching me in the process. The paroxysmal episode did not last long and ended as abruptly as it had begun. She crawled back onto the couch and slumped down in exhaustion.

We sat silently for several minutes. When she finally regained her faculties, she seemed confused and had no recollection of the harrowing event.

A skeptic might argue that my patient simply experienced a psychological condition known as a dissociative episode, which is known to occur in some patients who have a significant trauma history. While I concur that this is entirely possible, the fact that none of her family or friends had ever witnessed her having a dissociative episode previously would support an argument against this possibility. Knowing that trauma is a well-known open door for malevolent spiritual entities, I believe it is also possible that, in an emotionally charged therapy session, I had witnessed a rare phenomenon: the manifestation of an unseen spiritual entity.

True cases of demonic influence, or the much rarer phenomenon of demon possession, involve certain characteristics that have not been witnessed in people suffering from mental illness or acute intoxication by a mind-altering substance. These include psychic abilities, enabling them to reveal hidden knowledge; an unusually strong aversion to anything holy; openly blasphemous tirades or physical aggression; the ability to speak foreign languages unknown to the individual; and abnormal physical abilities, such as superhuman strength, wall climbing, seemingly impossible bodily contortions, and even, as documented in rare instances, levitation.

While these phenomena are rarely discussed in professional circles, and even less commonly in public, I have experienced so many other examples in my twenty-eight-year career of what I believe to be patients afflicted by undue influence from spiritual enemies that space does not allow me to elaborate in this context. But mental health practitioners and emergency department physicians are not alone. These phenomena are even more commonly witnessed by evangelical missionaries serving in countries or regions where the predominant religious practices are pagan in nature, such as voodoo, black magic, and witchcraft. Many traditional religious clergy and law enforcement officers in the United States have reportedly witnessed these phenomena so often that it is common knowledge in some circles, although, again, rarely spoken of publicly.

The Need for Patients to Acknowledge Spiritual Warfare

As a psychiatrist and physician, I believe it is paramount that patients not only accept but embrace the reality of unseen spiritual warfare, because it is the only view that helps make sense of the suffering, trouble, and evil we see in this world. Likewise, it is the only worldview that will give patients the tools to respond most appropriately and effectively to the injustice they experience in this world, instead of solely blaming God, others, or themselves.

Acceptance is an important concept in the field of medicine in general, and in psychiatry in particular. For example, it is widely recognized as the final stage of the grieving process, first proposed by psychiatrist Dr. Elisabeth Kübler-Ross in her 1969 book titled *On Death and Dying*. Furthermore, acceptance is the foundation of the first of the Twelve Steps widely employed in the field of addiction medicine, without which, denial or minimization often persists, hindering recovery. In order for the proposed principles of Ruachiatry to be successfully implemented in clinical practice, patients, likewise, must first accept the veiled reality of the spiritual world and then learn to fight and ultimately win these unseen battles with malevolent forces. As much as patients prefer peace, they simply cannot remain neutral in this invisible war. They must either side with the kingdom of God or the kingdom of darkness. They must either become soldiers fighting the good fight or unwitting "children of disobedience," destined to become casualties in the cosmic war. This news is a critical forewarning because, as Miguel de Cervantes said, "Forewarned is forearmed; to be prepared is half the victory."[8]

3

A SKEPTIC EXPERIENCES
THE SUPERNATURAL

The [spiritually ignorant] fool has said in his heart,
"There is no God."

—PSALMS 14:1 (AMP)

A Calling from a Young Age

I had a deep sense of a calling from a very young age. I do not think that I am unique in this respect, as I have come to believe that all humans are created with unique abilities and characteristics specifically tailored by our Creator to fulfill his purpose for our lives. However, not everyone hears the call. I believe this is because people either do not have their antennae up, they are tuned to the incorrect frequency and thus hear the much louder call of the world system and their own fleshly desires, or are simply not listening, often due to distraction or outright refusal to do so. The one who calls most often does so in a still, small voice, as he did to the Israelite prophet Elijah.[1] However, God certainly can and does at times shout, getting our attention by means of adversity in our lives, as he did in the dramatic case of blinding the Apostle Paul on the road to Damascus.[2]

I feel blessed to have been born in the United States to loving and highly educated parents, who provided me with a nurturing, supportive home environment and opportunities for growth and learning throughout my formative years. I vividly remember between the ages of three and four watching an old 1970s TV series titled *Emergency!* and being fascinated by the brave men and women who acted as paramedics, firefighters, doctors, and nurses to save others' lives. For some reason, the role of the doctor deeply resonated with me, and I decided at a very young age that was what I wanted to be when I grew up.

Early on, people noted that I had a precocious intellect and often preferred to converse with adults rather than other children. My family valued education, and I came from a long line of highly educated professionals, including a founding father and signer of the US Constitution. I performed well academically and became fascinated with science and nature, especially the cosmos, filled with stars, moons, and planets. Starting in seventh grade, I attended a prestigious Roman Catholic college preparatory private school, where religion and theology were a mandatory part of the curriculum. Like many Americans, I grew up a nominal Christian, meaning our family identified as Christian but attended worship services irregularly. The Bible was a nice big book that was revered for some reason I didn't understand, and at home, it sat prominently on our bookshelf collecting dust.

I believed there was a God only because authority figures told me so. Although I showed a natural aptitude for religious studies during high school, I dismissed the subject matter as unimportant because I felt it was nonacademic. I came to see science as the highest intellectual pursuit, and my childhood aspirations to study medicine began to crystallize. The church my family attended would occasionally refer to Jesus as "savior," but I recall being genuinely puzzled about what I needed to be saved from. I felt as though my life were charmed, and I was a healthy, well-behaved, high-achieving, conscientious firstborn child with a bright future. Why would I need saving from that?

Pride and the Illusion of Control

My spiritual state at the time calls to mind an encounter Jesus had with a "rich, young ruler," as described in the Gospel of Mark. The Greek word used there by Mark for *rich* refers to something useful or needed, not necessarily money. At the age of eighteen, I certainly was not rich monetarily, although my father, as a dentist who owned a successful private practice, did provide us a comfortable lifestyle. I was graciously given the many blessings in my life, and it made no logical sense for me to be prideful; I had no hand in procuring any of these blessings. Nevertheless, I was prideful and self-absorbed at that stage in my life, and I possessed an attitude of arrogance and entitlement rather than one of gratitude and thanksgiving.

Because of the natural gifts that I had been given, a keen intellect, and a strong work ethic, by the time I entered college, my confidence had blossomed into outright arrogance. I acted as any natural young man would be expected to act in the absence of a regenerate spirit; I lived to pursue the pleasures that the world has to offer—what the Bible calls the lust of the flesh, the lust of the eyes, and the pride of life. If there were a God, he seemed distant and uninterested, and I reserved my perceived right to call on him when needed, almost like one would a genie. Aimlessly following the crowd along the broad path of least resistance, I genuinely felt as though nothing I wanted was out of my reach.

In retrospect, I am ashamed to say that I was beginning to act as my own god, believing I had total and omnipotent control over my life and my destiny. Having yet to face any significant adversity whatsoever in my young life, I was set up to learn the hard biblical lessons that pride does indeed go before the Fall and that "God opposes the proud but shows favor to the humble."[3]

Academic Setbacks

I began my college career on the premed track, and the first semester, I took a very rigorous course load, choosing to take more credit hours than my advisor recommended. In spite of this, I indulged in a robust social life, leading to me contracting a mononucleosis infection a month into the first semester. Initially, I thought the sore throat I experienced was simple pharyngitis, so I did not seek a medical evaluation. By the time I did seek treatment, at the student health center on campus, I was quite ill with significant lethargy, high fever, difficulty swallowing, profound weight loss, and an enlarged liver and spleen. My case was so advanced by that time that the doctors decided to admit me to the hospital. I was too weak to walk and stayed there for nearly two weeks.

Because I had a heavy course load, with difficult subjects, and had missed so many class sessions, my premed academic advisor recommended that I drop some classes or withdraw from the semester altogether. Concerned that either of those options would get me off the premed track, I made the unwise choice to continue with all of my classes—which led me to getting Cs in biology and chemistry and logging a 2.79 GPA. I was devastated. I had never gotten a C on a paper or test, let alone as a final grade for a course.

When I met with my premed advisor at the end of the semester, he looked at me solemnly across his cluttered mahogany desk. "Tom," he said, "you're obviously not going to medical school, so you need to start thinking about another major."

Not exactly the encouragement I was hoping for. Indignant, I told him in no uncertain terms that I would be going to medical school, that I would be looking for another advisor, and that I would return to see him in three years after gaining my acceptance.

The following semester I performed better academically, and with hard work and perseverance, I maintained close to a 4.0 GPA for the rest of my college career. I had overcome the early adversity in my collegiate journey and was now poised to be a strong candidate for acceptance to medical school. Or so I thought.

The Crushing Rejection

In the fall of my senior year in college, it was time for me to start applying to medical schools. Generally speaking, the process is ultra-competitive, and one has the best chance of being accepted to a public medical school in his state of residence. In public state medical schools, usually 10 percent or fewer of the incoming first-year class are from out of state. Hence, an average state medical school can be nearly as difficult for nonresidents of that state to gain admittance to as an Ivy League program. I decided to spread my net broadly throughout the southeast, where I wanted to eventually settle. I also applied to some private medical colleges in the eastern United States.

My decision not to apply to my state's newest medical school—which was geared toward rural medicine—was based on the fact that, the previous summer, I had worked at a prestigious hospital in Atlanta with a team of cardiothoracic surgeons. As an immature and carnally minded twenty-one-year-old, I was attracted to this field because of the power that the surgeons wielded, the Porsches that they drove, and the thrill of working with someone's life hanging in the balance. It had nothing to do with any altruistic interest in helping my fellow man.

Early in the fall, during my senior year of undergraduate studies, I went back to the premed advisor who had told me three years earlier that I would not be going to medical school. He said that the premed committee would highly recommend me for admittance to medical school and that I should have no trouble getting into my state's public medical college, where I had decided I wanted to receive my medical education. As expected, in October, I was granted an interview there. It went very well, and so did the one that followed it. The second and final interview was with a physician, and we hit it off personally. By the end of the interview, we cut through all the pretense and talked more about baseball and football than medicine. He told me that he umpired in his spare time for fun, and I informed him that I, too, had once umpired—for Little League Baseball. The doctor seemed thrilled and said he hoped to see me there next year. He asked me to call him so we could ump together. I felt confident that I would get an acceptance letter soon thereafter.

But it was not to be. I rarely received mail in college, and would usually check my post office box only about once a week. However, because I was expecting a letter of acceptance from the medical college any day, I walked from my room on the fourth floor of the dorm across the quad to check my box every single day. Despite having earned excellent grades at a very academically rigorous university, scoring well on the MCAT, and receiving excellent letters of recommendation for medical school, by the time Christmas break rolled around, I had gotten rejection letters from all but two of the fifteen schools to which I had applied. Early on, I was not alarmed, because I didn't expect to be admitted to a state school where I was not a resident. However, when my fraternity brothers began fishing the rejection letters out of the trash can and posting them on the bulletin board in the lodge for all to see, my inflated ego began to deflate.

By February, I began to worry that I still had not heard from my state's medical college, but I had received a letter requesting a personal interview at a private medical school in my state. Those interviews also went well, but even though three generations of my father's side of the family had graduated from dental school there, I was not interested in attending, because the college was in the middle of a large city. By the time I got my undergraduate degree in May, I still had not heard from either of the two remaining schools. My confidence was waning, and doubt crept in for the first time. Soon thereafter, I received news that I had been placed on the wait-list at the private medical school. There was still hope, though, as I was awaiting my acceptance from the state medical college.

After graduation, I went back to my parents' home for the summer. I checked the mailbox every day for the acceptance letter from my state's medical college. Finally, one muggy Georgia afternoon in late June, when I slapped a leash on my trusty cocker spaniel, Murph, and headed down the hill to our mailbox, I found a thin envelope in it from my state's medical college. My heart fluttered as I opened the letter on the spot, knowing deep down that a thin envelope could only spell bad news. As I read the four-line rejection, my heart sank to the pit of my stomach, and I literally felt weak in the knees, as if someone had knocked my legs out from under me. My head was swimming. My thoughts were swirling. My world was caving in around me, as everything I had worked so hard for and felt I had earned was suddenly taken from me for inexplicable reasons.

Collision Course with a Supernatural Power

I had wanted to be a doctor almost since infancy. What was I going to do now? I froze there in front of the mailbox, with tears streaming down my face. I didn't know what to do. I couldn't go back to the house yet, because my parents were there. I didn't feel like dealing with their reactions yet. I decided I would just walk around the neighborhood with Murph and try to regain my composure.

I had not walked very far when I stopped suddenly in the middle of the street. I was hurt, confused, and genuinely perplexed about why this had happened. Although I did not know it at the time, I have come to learn that God is not the author of confusion, but the Devil certainly is. Thirty-three years later, I realize that this was an instance of what the Apostle Paul described in 1 Corinthians 10:13 as *peirasmos*, a Greek word meaning "adversity sent by God to test one's character, faith, and holiness." Satan wants to turn these tests of righteousness into temptations to solicit evil. How was I going to respond? Would I pass the most difficult test so far in my young life?

Out of desperation and having nowhere else to turn, I cried out to God as, once again, tears streamed down my face. But this time I was angry. In retrospect, I am embarrassed that I addressed the Almighty in such a disrespectful way.

It went something like this: *What the hell? I've worked all my life for this, and you are going to take it from me? Really? I earned this—it's not fair! You know what, I'm not even sure if I believe in you. What kind of god would do this to one of his children anyway? If you are real and you are who you say you are, then I need you to show me right now. I'm not saying you need to grant me entrance into medical school, but you need to reveal yourself to me, and you need to show me what you want me to do with my life. If you do that, I promise I will follow you the rest of my days.*

I was just another doubting Thomas, demanding proof but not actually expecting any response.

Immediately, an unseen presence surrounded me. It felt as though time stood still. Then an inexplicable feeling of peace permeated the air around me. But what happened next really blew my mind. Words do not do it justice, but I will try to describe it anyway.

Unseen arms wrapped around me, tightly pulling me toward an invisible bosom.

I was enveloped by indescribable peace and love. I felt a reassurance that all was well and was going to continue to be well, despite the adverse circumstances. I believed it without question at the time because of the incredibly intense emotions involved in the experience, along with the inexplicable sensation of touch. I was overwhelmed. I don't know how else to explain it except to say that it was truth, without any doubt involved whatsoever.

When the embrace ended, I still felt an otherworldly presence that was comforting beyond measure. I decided to continue on my approximately two-mile walk around the neighborhood with Murph before returning home. When I arrived home and told my parents of the news, they were as crestfallen as I was. Their natural inclination was to do something, and so they immediately started discussing ideas to contact people and pull strings to get me off the wait-list at my state's private medical school.

"How can you be so calm?" my dad asked me.

I did not think they would understand. Maybe they would even think I had gone crazy—so I did not tell them about my supernatural visitation. After several days of my parents' behind-the-scenes efforts, it seemed that my best chance was to have an interview with the dean of the newer medical school in my state—the one geared toward rural medicine that I hadn't applied to because of my interest in cardiothoracic surgery and my overconfidence that I would gain admission to one of the two other medical schools in my state.

It turned out that my mom knew the dean of that medical school, so she called him to discuss my situation. He told her that he could not guarantee they could admit me, but he was kind enough to arrange an interview with me. It seemed there was hope.

Several days later, I got dressed up in my Sunday best to drive the hundred-mile trek south to speak with the dean. I vividly recall

lingering on the couch in our living room despite my mom's pleadings to leave early so that I would not be late. Somehow, I had this
strange sense that this was not the way to go, but I was willing to
pursue this path because my parents had worked hard to open this
door of opportunity for me.

"Tommy, you need to leave now!" my mom finally barked at me.

Something inside was telling me to linger a little bit longer for
reasons I didn't understand. When I finally made my way to the
back door of our house, I kissed my parents goodbye. I had my hand
on the doorknob when the phone on the laundry room wall rang. I
stopped in my tracks as my mom answered it.

"Yes. Yes, he's right here," she stammered with a puzzled look on
her face. "It's for you."

"Who is it?" I whispered.

"It's for you!" Mom replied impatiently, thrusting the phone in
my direction.

On the other end of the line was the dean of admissions for the
private medical college I had ultimately hoped to attend. He was
calling to ask if I would be willing to have my name removed from
the wait-list and officially accept a position for the first-year medical school class. I was floored.

"Yes, sir!" I replied.

The dean gave me instructions on next steps and informed me
that there was not much time, as classes began the following week.
When I hung up the phone and told my parents the news, jubila-
tion ensued like I have rarely seen from them.

Humility and the Path Forward

For the first time in my young life, all traces of arrogance in me
were gone. I had been humbled in a completely inexplicable and
unexpected way, and now I was genuinely grateful.

Because humility is the prerequisite to any genuine spiritual journey, it is not difficult to see why many people, like me, who have character traits of self-sufficiency, pride, and even outright arrogance, are blinded to spiritual truths and tend to lack consistent spiritual practices in their lives. Jesus commented on this observation following his conversation with the rich young ruler I mentioned earlier. This blessed young man chose not to follow Jesus, because Jesus asked him to first sell all he owned. Tragically, the young man calculated the cost Jesus required and decided it was too high. He chose fleeting, material blessings over eternal, spiritual blessings.

Jesus looked around and said to his disciples, "How hard it is for the rich to enter the kingdom of God!"[4]

It was indeed difficult for a man of wealth, status, and distinction to voluntarily surrender his riches and rank and all that made life worthwhile to him in order to openly follow the increasingly despised Jesus and his motley crew. Despite my irreverence in the midst of my uncertainty about my medical school admission, I can now see that I had still responded with surrender. In my frustration, anger, and confusion, I was still effectively saying to God, "I'm mad and don't know what you want me to do now, but if you will show me, I will do it." He physically embraced me and then orchestrated my circumstances to grant me what I wanted most. I have come to understand that he granted me this not because it was my desire but because it was his desire for me; he was just waiting for me to accept that reality.

Exercising My Responsibility to Discover the Truth

After this encounter, I felt a great sense of responsibility and became willing to leave everything behind in order to live up to this calling. Now I indeed knew that the unseen spiritual world was a reality and that there was some unseen higher power who could somehow hear the thoughts I silently prayed. Even so, I still did not know God as I know him today.

When I began medical school, I was absolutely fascinated by the intricacies of the human body, right down to the complexities within every single one of its thirty trillion cells. There were so many small things that could go awry during embryological development and during the life cycle that it was a wonder to me that there was not *more* disease and death. The complexities of the human body left me with no doubt that there had to be a designer. Cells did not differentiate and develop specialized functions from evolution, I reasoned.

I was now ready to explore different religious faiths in a quest to find God. For thousands of years, there has been evidence that nearly all cultures and civilizations of the world have believed in an unseen spiritual realm. Most of these worshipped gods or a god, but I couldn't help but wonder which one was the true God. I needed to find out, especially if I intended to live up to my end of the bargain I had made with my unseen benefactor. I began my pursuit by mapping out a reading plan of the major texts of world religions. Since I was raised a Christian in a Western culture and educated at a Catholic school, I made a conscious decision to explore Christianity last, due to any potential inherent bias I might have.

When I studied in the evenings after class at medical school, I would take along whichever of these sacred texts I happened to be reading at the time to peruse during study breaks. I am certain that classmates saw it as odd, but I was on a relentless mission to find answers to my spiritual questions and then to wholeheartedly serve the being who had rescued me.

I began by reading the Hindu Vedas and Upanishads followed by the Muslim Quran. I then moved to the Buddhist Tipitaka, followed by the Tanakh of Judaism. I discovered there was wisdom and truth in all of these texts, and I gained a newfound understanding and respect for why millions of people found them helpful. But I found problems and questions within many of these texts, whether it was internal inconsistencies or purported truths that defied logic or scientific evidence. For example, I grappled with the fact that the Hindu Vedas describe the Earth as a convex disc that rests on the backs of eight elephants (*diggajas*), which stand on a cosmic turtle (*adi-kurma*) that, in turn, rests on the 1,000-headed serpent of time (*ananta-sesha*).

Death of a Boy and Rebirth of a Man

Finally, it was time to turn to the Christian Bible. Believe it or not, I had never read the entire Bible, only selected portions of it for academic reasons during Catholic school and for a college class. I was dumbfounded. I came to see it as the only text that accurately described human beings, creation, and the world in which we live. I came to realize God's plan for the salvation of all mankind through the substitutionary, sacrificial death of his son Jesus. For the first time, I realized that I was a sinner without hope and in desperate need of a savior.

My life was forever changed in early 1993, when I prayed to accept Jesus Christ's death on the cross as payment for my sin debt, which I owed to God due to both my inherited sinful nature and the multitude of actual sins of commission, omission, thought, and deed that I had perpetrated throughout my life. I now identified the third person of the Trinity, the Holy Spirit, as the unseen benevolent presence I had experienced after receiving my letter of rejection from medical school. I was thrilled to learn that upon my profession of faith, that very same Spirit would come to live inside of me and become a life-giving Spirit, essentially reviving the dead spirit I had received at birth as a consequence of mankind's original sin.[5] I have never gotten over my experience on the street in front of my childhood home nor my eventual surrender to the Lordship of Jesus, and I pray that I never will.

Illumination of the Less-Trodden Path

I moved forward in my medical studies, keeping an open mind about which area of medicine I wanted to pursue. I still felt like surgery was the right route for me, but for some reason, I had an inner conflict about this. Pursuit of a career in surgery seemed to be a desire from my old life that I'd left behind when I surrendered to God's plan for me. To my other surprise, when I did a rotation in psychiatry during my third year of medical school, I both very much enjoyed it and seemed to have a natural aptitude for it. I did not want this to be the case. I erroneously and naively felt that only weirdos or damaged people looking to fix themselves would enter this field as a career. Once I completed several surgery rotations, I realized that the training and lifestyle of many of the subspecialties in which I was interested might not afford me the time I desired to devote to my family and to pursue my interests outside of medicine.

During my fourth and final year of medical school, I began to seriously entertain psychiatry as a career option. When I discussed this with my parents, my proposal was not initially well received. However, my girlfriend at the time, who would eventually become my wife, encouraged me. I was intrigued by the fact that psychiatry afforded the physician an opportunity to work with not only sickness of the body but also sickness of the soul. The ultimate catalyst came when I read a book by renowned Viennese psychiatrist Viktor

Frankl, MD, titled *The Doctor and the Soul*, which delves deeper into this fascinating reality. Frankl was a Jew born in Austria who lived through the horrors of two world wars, spending three years in four Nazi concentration camps, including Auschwitz, where more than 1.2 million Jews were murdered. Frankl lost both parents, his brother, and his wife in these camps. Having survived this evil himself, Frankl went on to write with great authority about finding meaning in life, especially amid horrendous suffering and injustice.

After bathing the matter in much prayer and talking with several medical school advisors, I decided to take the plunge into this mysterious field of medicine that addresses both body and soul. It seemed as though I was taking the road less traveled, but it just felt right. I have never regretted my decision—not for a second—because I believe God led me to it and was gracious enough to grant me the privilege of practicing a profession where I found the intersection of what I was naturally good at, a subject I was interested in, and work I enjoyed. Like Jonah, I learned that you can't outrun God, and like Adam and Eve, I also learned that you cannot hide from him. God is indeed the hound of heaven, as described in Francis Thompson's famous poem, who is relentless in hunting down his children.[6] I am so very grateful to the loving, patient God who met me where I was: a self-willed young man facing rejection, loss, and the depths of despair on that lonely street in Georgia back in 1992. He had seemingly given me the desire of my heart when I responded to my trial by surrendering to his will, and I was excited to follow him and see his plan for my life unfold.

4

A BRIEF SPIRITUAL HISTORY OF THE WORLD

History is a story written by the finger of God.
—C. S. LEWIS

Introduction: A Spiritual Lens on History

I love history, probably because it is the story of human beings, and I have dedicated my professional life to understanding their minds—how they think, what motivates them, and what makes them anxious or depressed. Not surprisingly, I chose the field of history as a major for my undergraduate college degree. However, it was not until I later came to have faith in God that I realized that, while he grants humans free will, God is sovereign and will accomplish his will and plans with or without the aid of his human family.[1]

Hence, history is really God's story. Therefore, seeing it through a spiritual lens is a vital concept lost on the academic world, in which scholars tend to stay on their own turf in their own backyards, rarely integrating accumulated knowledge from disparate fields of study, such as theology, psychology, or history. In an effort at integration, we must have a framework, and I have chosen the Judeo-Christian Bible as the reference point, given the fact that it is both the oldest and most widely read book considered holy Scripture. This chapter will, therefore, present a very limited overview of how mankind's history intersects with what the Old and New Testaments teach about the history of spiritual beings and the spiritual world. While there is no great predictor of human behavior, I learned in my psychiatric training at Duke that the best predictor of future behavior is past behavior. Hence, it could be a vital part of our battle plan in the invisible war to understand how the enemy operated in times past. After all, as Winston Churchill famously asserted in a 1948 speech to the British House of Commons, "Those who fail to learn from history are doomed to repeat it."

The times in which we live have been called the "age of anxiety," and as a psychiatrist, I can attest to the fact that anxiety is not only extremely common but also increasing in prevalence. I believe this is in large part due to the fact that many people today look around at the unsettling circumstances of life, such as rapid technological change and social upheaval, instead of looking up to the one who is in ultimate control of it all. It is all about our perspective. I believe that if people can fully grasp the reality that there exist unseen evil forces that attack the purposes of God, both on a global and personal level, their ability to cope with life stressors will improve drastically.

On a national level, we should not be surprised when we observe escalating crime, violence, disease, pandemics, social discord, economic crises, environmental catastrophes, and political divisiveness, among a host of other problems. Although the theory of evolution has erroneously programmed us to believe that circumstances should be getting progressively better, the observable scientific law of entropy clearly displays the fact that things are actually descending into a progressively greater state of chaos across the board. In this world, we will have trouble, so expect it.[2] I am not suggesting that we should be negative and cynical, but rather that we should be vigilant and not caught off guard when adversity inevitably strikes.

The same holds true for adversity in our personal lives.

As difficult as it may be to fathom, God decreed plans and a purpose for each of our individual lives before we were ever conceived, and he promises to work all things, even adverse circumstances, together for the good of everyone who loves him and is called according to his purposes.[3]

While it is true that bad things happen in life, more often than most people realize, there is a hidden hand orchestrating some adversities in our lives in an attempt to thwart God's purpose and plan for us. If we are walking according to God's will and plan for our lives, we will be attacked by our enemies. As we shall see, our enemies not only know God's plan—albeit incompletely—for mankind over vast periods of time in human history, but our demonic foes also know God's plans for us as individuals. Often, the precise focus of their attacks inadvertently unveils God's plans for our individual lives. The greater the attack, the greater God's plans for us, in all likelihood. We must not only expect these attacks but also engage in a rigorous examination of their nature in order to illuminate the unique plans God has sovereignly appointed for our lives.

The Origins of the Cosmic Battle

As in any story, we must start at the beginning. The book of beginnings, the book of Genesis in the Bible, is a logical reference point. Said by scholars to have been written about 3,500 years ago by Moses, Genesis tells of a self-existent, omnipotent God who created mankind in his own image for his own pleasure. He then gave mankind dominion and the title deed to the earth, a realm that initially overlapped with heaven and therefore gave humans unfettered access to God. This Supreme spiritual being existed among a host of lesser spiritual beings he had created, called *elohim*, or what we call *angels* today. God's goal was for his two families, his immortal spiritual family (angels) and his earthly physical family (humans), to peacefully coexist and work toward bringing about his will in each of these two realms. Both families were created to be immortal, but then something happened that changed their destinies.

One of these elohim, who was said to be the greatest of God's created spiritual family, did not approve of God's created physical beings and pridefully saw himself as superior. The idea of serving these inferior creatures, made from the dust of the earth, was likely abhorrent to him.[4] This anointed and gifted cherub saw himself as a leader to be praised rather than a humble servant. So, he hatched a plan to get rid of his inferior physical rivals.

The First Rebellion: The Fall of Man

This *nachash*, or *shining one*, often translated as *serpent* in modern translations of the Bible, knew that taking matters into his own hands and killing the humans directly would be a clear affront to God himself, holding grave consequences. So, this adversary used lies and trickery to entice mankind to rebel and doubt both God's Word and his goodness, invoking God's judgment on them—death. Essentially, God, being just and righteous, would have no choice but to inflict holy justice on his beloved physical creatures, whom he'd made in his image. The adversary's brilliant plan was to have God himself do the killing, thus eliminating these inferior rivals.

This coup was successful in that the nachash did successfully trick his physical siblings and wrestle away the title deed to the earth. But his days were numbered. Satan fired the first shot in the war, but God's second shot was not the response his adversary was expecting. Satan, in his pride, had grossly underestimated God, who, being omnipotent and omniscient, foreknew Satan's plans but had kept secret his own counterplan.[5] Although mankind had no means of access to the holy Creator nor any hope of restoration, God displayed his love for us by initiating a plan to rescue humanity and the physical universe from the now inevitable divine judgment for evil. Shockingly, God himself would become human, enter the physical world, and pay the penalty due for mankind's transgression.

When God revealed his secret plan to delay judgment on the physical world and give mankind an opportunity for redemption in Genesis, Chapter 3, Satan was furious. God announced to the rebellious cherub that from then on there would be ongoing war between him and mankind, and between Satan's offspring and the woman's offspring.

And I will cause hostility between you and the woman, and between your offspring and her offspring. He will strike your head, and you will strike his heel.[6]

Satan is one of the elohim, a created spiritual being lacking the ability to procreate. So how can he have offspring? The answer likely lies in the fact that Satan roams the earth looking for willing humans—who are sold out to their carnal desires and to the world system he governs—to join his family as adopted rebellious sons and daughters, just as God adopts willing human sons and daughters into his family, if they choose to accept Jesus's death as payment for their sins.

Until his future day of judgment, this powerful cherub called Satan is god of this world, a ruthless king of a seized kingdom who subjects its rightful rulers to a shortened life filled with futility, toil, hardship, disease, and, ultimately, physical death. Satan indeed gained the whole world that he sought, but he lost his soul in the process. His ultimate destiny is to be confined to the hell created for him and the other fallen angels who followed his rebellion. It is of vital importance to note that this place of eternal fire and torment was created only for the fallen angels, not for man. All mankind had to do to avoid this fate was simply acknowledge and gratefully accept God's sacrifice for their sin and then embrace the faith to follow him and his plan for their lives. This is still all that mankind has to do. The choice is simple: Follow the god of this world or the omnipotent creator God, Yahweh. The choice carries eternal implications.

Mankind's aversion to and fear of death is rooted in the fact that we have a deep primordial sense that the seeming finality of death is at its essence just not right, not the way things were originally intended to be, because "God has planted eternity in the human heart."[7] We were created to live forever, not die, and somewhere, deep down inside, we know it. As C. S. Lewis said, "If we find ourselves with a desire that nothing in this world can satisfy, the most probable explanation is that we were made for another world."[8]

Access to that world vanished at the Fall, but God promises to restore it one day. Until then, "The creation looks forward to the day when it will join God's children in glorious freedom from death and decay."[9] In addition to a cosmic war, another consequence of the rebellion in the spiritual realm was that a border—what Scripture calls a "veil"—was placed between heaven and earth, only to be partially opened at specific points in the nation of Israel's history to foreshadow the day it will be fully reopened when God restores the link between the two kingdoms of his spiritual and physical families. This veil is to protect us from a holy, sinless God, who is pure light. Otherwise, mankind would perish in the presence of this consuming fire.

The enemy takes advantage of this veil, essentially using it as camouflage, to conduct his military campaigns stealthily in the invisible spiritual realm that surrounds our physical reality. As Charles Baudelaire wrote in his short story "The Generous Gambler": "The Devil's cleverest wile is to make men believe that he does not exist."[10] His hiding behind the veil, pulling the strings of history like the Wizard of Oz, makes it easy for scientifically minded men and women to dismiss the idea of a devil being behind much of the injustice, sickness, destruction, violence, and death in the world. Since we cannot visualize, examine, test, and retest the supposed phenomenon, it is not scientific and is, therefore, reasoned to not be objectively "true." Faith is wrongly viewed by many modern scientists as the blind superstition of uneducated people who are desperate to find some meaning in their brief lives on this planet. This conclusion is just what Satan desires.

There is another plan of the enemy at work beyond the denial that he and his army exist in the first place.

The Second Rebellion: The Rise of Evil Before the Flood

Once the fallen angels learned of God's plan to one day bring forth a human savior from the seed of Eve, they hatched a plot to prevent this by corrupting the human genome so that mankind would no longer bear the image of their Creator.

Genesis Chapter 6 describes a second rebellion by members of God's spiritual family, a peculiar incursion in which a group of rebel angels went after "strange flesh" and took for themselves wives among human women. Somehow, the human women they chose gave birth to hybrids called *Nephilim* (a Hebrew term meaning "fallen ones"), many of whom became mighty men of renown, giants such as Og of Bashan, Goliath, and the Sumerian hero Gilgamesh. According to non-scriptural Jewish texts from the Second Temple period (536 BC to 70 AD), such as the *First Book of Enoch*, the *Book of Giants*, and the *Book of Jubilees*, these half-breed fallen ones were aggressive and bloodthirsty, causing chaos on earth. This chaos grew so extreme that God became sorry he had ever made mankind and decided to destroy the world with a great flood. Satan had almost succeeded in annihilating the seed of the woman, but sovereign God chose to start over, sparing eight people—a righteous man of pure lineage, Noah, and his family.

The Third Rebellion: Tower of Babel and the Division of Nations

After the flood, God commanded mankind to spread out and repopulate the entire earth, but it didn't take long for mankind to disobey again. Satan influenced Noah's great-grandson, the mighty man Nimrod, to build great cities for the people to populate rather than spreading out as the animals had. Nimrod was a satanically influenced rebel against God who became the world's first emperor and a model for future antichrists throughout history to follow.

According to both Jewish and Islamic traditions, Nimrod was bent on revenge against God for the great flood, and he was the first king to ever wear a crown.[11] The Jewish historian Flavius Josephus stated that Nimrod had such "contempt of God" that he "gradually changed the government into tyranny, seeing no other way of turning men from the fear of God."[12] This mighty self-proclaimed king built his kingdom in the land of Babylonia and founded the city of Babylon and its counterfeit religious system, described in the Bible as a *harlot*.[13]

According to Genesis, under Nimrod's rule, the people built the great tower at Babel, they said, to "make us famous and keep us from being scattered all over the world."[14] Nimrod attempted to unite the world and to exalt man by building a tower, a gate to God. Like Satan before him, Nimrod aspired to "ascend to heaven" and make himself like the Most High. God judged this idolatry by scattering the people all over the earth and confusing their language, as described in the Bible: "When the Most High divided the nations, when he separated the sons of Adam, he set the bounds of the nations, according to the number of the angels of God. And his people Jacob [the ancient Hebrew nation] became the portion of the Lord, Israel was the line of his inheritance."[15]

When God divided mankind into seventy nations at the Tower of Babel, he apportioned oversight of the nations to certain elohim, giving them varying levels of authority. For himself, God chose Abraham to be the father of the future nation of Israel and the archangel Michael as its spiritual overseer. Ever since then, Satan has placed in the hearts of carnal men the dream to once again unite the entire world under one government with one apostate religion and one satanically possessed dictator in order to fight against God and his people. There is continual spiritual warfare between the holy angels and the numerous fallen angels who have been given dominion over the nations of this world.

Israel: God's Chosen Nation in the Battle

God's rebellious spiritual family learned more of his plan when God announced his covenant with Abraham about 4,000 years ago. Through God's blessing of Abraham and his descendants, the whole earth would be blessed, since the Savior would ultimately come from his lineage.[16] Members of God's rebellious spiritual family then came up with a new tactic: annihilate the Jewish race and all descendants of Abraham so that the Savior could not be born.

Satan first tempted Abraham to lay with his Egyptian slave Hagar in order to bear him a son, since his wife Sarah was barren. Satan hoped Ishmael's birth would dilute the seed, but this plan was thwarted when Isaac was later miraculously born to Abraham and Sarah in their old age.[17]

Later, when Isaac's son Jacob stole his elder brother Esau's birthright, Satan likely shot some fiery arrows Esau's way, inflaming his anger into a murderous rage that prompted him to hunt his brother, who had fled into the wilderness. But God supernaturally protected Jacob from both Esau and surrounding nations and even eventually influenced the brothers to reconcile.[18] After sending peace offerings to Esau, Jacob had a wrestling match with an angel of the Lord, who renamed him "Israel." His twelve sons became the fathers of the Jewish people,[19] and Satan's plan to destroy the seed of Abraham was thwarted again.

Satan attempted to destroy Abraham's seed yet again when the nation of Israel was held captive in the land of Egypt, between approximately 1800 and 1400 BC. To prevent the Israelites from growing in number and rebelling, the pharaoh issued an order that all newborn Hebrew males be drowned in the Nile River. But the Hebrew baby Moses was providentially spared when he was rescued from the Nile by a member of the pharaoh's family.[20] The lineage was preserved, and Moses eventually became the nation's deliverer, chosen by God to lead their exodus from Egypt.

As the Israelites wandered in the desert and eventually marched toward the Promised Land of Canaan, many surrounding nations and peoples also attempted to annihilate them, starting with the Amalekites. Canaan, too, was filled with adversaries, giant genetically tainted descendants of the Nephilim, which is the reason God required their annihilation at the hands of his chosen people. The adversaries waged war with the Israelites for centuries, but as many of their enemies were annihilated, the tiny nation of Israel defied the odds and was preserved because God was with them.[21]

God had called for Abraham and, ultimately, Israel to be different from the nations—a light to the Gentiles, without any king but God himself. But Israel eventually rebelled against this intended theocratic government and wanted a human king, like the other nations. God turned them over to their desire but promised that one day the Messiah, a descendant of King David, would rule the entire united, redeemed world under a theocracy.[22]

When the enemies of God learned of this, they planned to bring about David's death. They first unsuccessfully used Goliath, then King Saul, in attempts to kill David. Later, Satan tempted him to commit adultery with Bathsheba, hoping that either her jealous husband, Uriah, or God himself would take David's life.

A final example of the enemy's attempt to prevent the Messiah's coming via genocide occurred in Persia around 500 BC, after the Persian king's evil vizier Haman commanded all the people to bow down to him. The book of Esther recounts how one righteous Jew, Mordecai, refused to do so, inciting Haman's wrath. In response to Mordecai's defiance, Haman devised a plan to exterminate all the Jews in the Persian empire, but the plot was foiled by the queen, Esther, who, unbeknownst to both the king and Haman, was a Jew herself.

The era that followed this is known as the "silent years," because no new prophets arose in Israel and no new scriptures were written during the 400 years leading up to the birth of Jesus.

The Birth of Christ: The Enemy's Desperate Counterattack

With the news of Jesus's birth, yet another strategy was needed by the enemy in the ongoing war between the fallen angels and God. Reminiscent of the pharaoh's edict approximately 1,500 years earlier, Satan convinced King Herod of Judaea to decree a slaughter of the innocent babies in Bethlehem under the age of two when he learned that Jesus had been born. However, after being supernaturally warned by an angel in a dream, Jesus's earthly father, Joseph, hurriedly left Bethlehem with his wife, Mary, and newborn son, narrowly escaping Herod's soldiers.[23]

About thirty years later, Satan went after Jesus again, this time in the Judaean wilderness in an unsuccessful effort to tempt him to stop following God's will. Defeated, Satan didn't launch an assault on Jesus again until a more opportune time: when he announced to his disciples that he would suffer and be killed but rise from the dead on the third day after his death. Hoping to discourage Jesus from honoring God's will by dying on the cross, Satan influenced the leader of Jesus's twelve apostles, Peter, to rebuke Jesus for saying that he would. This prompted Jesus's famous response: "Get thee behind me, Satan!"[24]

Realizing who Jesus was and that time to intervene was short, Satan then resolved that he would simply kill Jesus. The leader of the rebellious fallen angels brought about several storms when Jesus was at sea and influenced many to attempt to stone Jesus to death. But because Satan was neither omniscient nor omnipresent, he—unlike God—was bound by space, time, and limited knowledge. To come up with battle plans, Satan relied only on his experience, intellect, and knowledge of Jewish scriptures, with no help from the Holy Spirit for interpretation. Ultimately, at the crucifixion, God fooled Satan, who would have never stirred the religious and governmental authorities to put Jesus to death had he known what God was up to.

The Crucifixion: Satan's Defeat and the Birth of the Church

Although today, demons tend to hide and fight via guerrilla warfare, it was not always this way. Satan and his fallen angels once demanded worship. They would openly display their power to garner it and grant worldly favors and positions of power to their devotees. This changed after the crucifixion of Jesus Christ, when Jesus's act thwarted their plans and launched his counteroffensive through the devotion of his followers and the spread of his message to the world. The enemies of God receded into the spiritual realm behind the veil, where they continue to wreak havoc on the physical world in an attempt to thwart people from being saved from the fate that awaits them—death.

After his resurrection, Jesus appeared to his disciples for forty days and then ascended to heaven. He promised to send a spiritual guide—the Holy Spirit—to live within his followers and guide them as they traveled throughout the world spreading the good news of God's redemption offer to mankind. Jesus promised to return to his followers one day. Until that day, he instructed, they were to set up embassies in this physical world called *churches*, where his followers would serve as ambassadors of the truth in territory temporarily occupied by a foreign adversary.

The Church under Attack: From Persecution to Corruption

The enemy's new strategy then became to limit knowledge of God's redemptive offer and neutralize the efforts of his churches and followers throughout the world. Satan's efforts to limit the spread of the good news began from the very moment of Jesus's ascension, and they continue to this day. He immediately attempted to frighten the Apostles into silence, eventually having a hand in the execution of all but John. But even death could not stop the spread of the news. God's truth was loose and could not be contained, spreading out gradually to the entire known world, despite Satan's attempts to oppress believers and their efforts.

The early church was heavily persecuted by satanically influenced Roman emperors. Nero blamed the Christians for the burning of Rome and used captured believers as human torches. Other emperors crucified early Christians or compelled them to face lions or gladiators in the Colosseum for sport. Emperor Diocletian enacted violent persecution of early Christians in 303 and 304 AD, killing thousands and burning their scriptures. Amazingly, eight short years later, emperor Constantine saw a vision of the cross to which he credited his victory in the Battle of the Milvian Bridge. The event prompted him to issue the Edict of Milan the following year, an agreement to end the persecution of Christians in the Roman Empire. Christianity would become the official religion of the empire in 391 AD.

The Dark Ages: A Time of Spiritual Suppression

The fall of the Roman Empire in 476 heralded the beginning of the Middle Ages. This period was also called the Dark Ages, because during this time, Europe experienced significant political, economic, and social upheaval, and much of the knowledge and culture of the ancient world was lost. It was also dark because God's light of truth was significantly hindered. In many parts of Europe, there was a decline in urbanization and a decrease in trade and commerce, leading to a more localized and rural way of life. The period was characterized by frequent warfare, invasions by various tribes and other groups, and the rise of feudalism, a system of social hierarchy based on land ownership. Kings and other powerful nobles owned large tracts of land, which they would grant to their loyal vassals in exchange for military service or other forms of loyalty. These vassals, in turn, would sublet portions of their land to smaller landowners, who would pledge loyalty to them in return. Serfs were the lowest class in the feudal system. They were tied to the land and worked it for their lord in exchange for protection and the right to live on the land. Although not slaves, serfs were not free either. I have heard it said that serfs worked for their master for three months of the year.

The feudal system was hierarchical, with the king at the top and the serfs at the bottom. It was also decentralized, with power and authority resting in the hands of local lords rather than a centralized government. This made enforcing laws and maintaining order difficult and contributed to the instability and warfare that characterized much of medieval Europe. A precarious existence that relied on localized subsistence farming and afforded no possibility for the attainment of education or social advancement allowed the unseen enemy to further neutralize the effects of the Christian faith in Europe at this time. In spite of this, Christianity continued to spread. However, a new rival sprang up in the 600s and 700s—Islam, which largely relied upon the sword to gain converts, rather than proselytizing. Beginning in 1097 and lasting more than one hundred years, a number of crusades were waged between Christians and Muslims, with both sides committing atrocities in the name of their God.

At the beginning of the Middle Ages, the bishop of Rome, the Pope, had become the leading spokesman for the faith in Western Christendom. Over the next several centuries, the Roman Catholic Church became an increasingly hierarchical structure, with a central bureaucracy and the Pope as its head. As a result of the breakup of the Carolingian Empire in 843 AD, the tenth century saw a period of marked corruption within the church.

By 1231, the Roman Catholic Church under Gregory IX had established the papal Inquisition, ostensibly to combat heresies. The injustices and atrocities of the Inquisition are well documented, and local officials were empowered by the church to conduct inquisitions and trials and even to carry out capital punishment, if deemed necessary. In 1302, the Pope claimed supremacy over secular rulers and seven years later moved the papacy from Rome to Avignon, France.

From 1348 to 1351, the world saw the rise of the Black Death, the bubonic plague that killed nearly one-third of all Europeans, many of whom blamed the disease on the Avignon papacy. The plague thus indirectly led to a weakening of Roman authority in Western Europe, as evidenced by the Great Schism within the Catholic Church between 1378 and 1417, a tumultuous period when three men simultaneously claimed to be the legitimate Pope. I believe that the reduction of the population in Europe by forty million people and the greater centralization, bureaucratization, and secularization of the church over several centuries in the early Middle Ages, as well as the eventual weakening of the church's authority after the bubonic plague, were all designs by the unseen enemies.

Additionally, the spiritual enemies were able to limit access to the written Word of God in the Holy Bible to a select few for more than 1400 years. In 1371, English priest John Wycliffe stated that scripture should be made available to the people in their own language, an assertion that caused discord with the Roman Catholic Church. In 1408, it became illegal to translate or read the Bible in English without permission from a bishop. Ten years later, the Roman Catholic Church officially rejected Wycliffe's teachings and pronounced his follower Jan Hus of Bohemia a heretic, and they burned him at the stake. It wasn't until Johannes Gutenberg invented the printing press in 1440 that numerous copies of the Bible were able to be printed and distributed to people in their native tongues.

The Reformation: Breaking the Chains of Spiritual Control

The fifteenth-century faithful in Western Europe became increasingly soured by the church's widespread sale of *indulgences*, a payment purported by the church to reduce the punishment for sins, giving rise to anti-papal reformatory movements. In 1517, priest Martin Luther nailed his *Ninety-Five Theses* outlining necessary reforms of the Roman Catholic Church to the door of his church in Wittenberg, Germany, starting the Protestant Reformation. Faith in Christ alone, said the Reformers, saved one from the penalty of sin, not indulgences. Soon thereafter, in response to William Tyndale translating the Bible into English in 1525 and smuggling copies into England in sacks of corn, the unseen infernal forces worked behind the scenes to ensure Tyndale was stopped when he was burned at the stake in 1536.

Despite the constant counterattacks to the spread of God's good news, the Reformation and Protestant proliferation throughout Europe ensured that additional translations of the Bible were circulated. By the late 1600s and early 1700s, translated copies were so ubiquitous that the Catholic Church could no longer enforce edicts against them. It is no coincidence that as God's truth broke out and spread rapidly across the globe, freedom and human progress in art (the Renaissance), exploration (Columbus, Vasco da Gama, and Magellan's discoveries of new lands and establishment of colonial empires), and science (the Scientific Revolution, beginning in the sixteenth century, which brought about major advances in mathematics, physics, and other fields) seemed to follow. Pandora's box had been opened, and a new strategy was needed by the enemy again.

The Age of Reason: Science vs. Faith

Enter the Age of Reason, the Enlightenment, which promulgated the ideas of secular humanism, rationalism, empiricism, reason, and science.

The Enlightenment entailed a radical shift in values, ethics, morality, and faith that was formerly considered absolute. The spiritual contribution to illness became abrogated to the biological as the Roman Catholic Church's objections to human dissection loosened, enabling physicians to gain a greater understanding of the link between disease and anatomical anomalies. Likewise, influential works of the sixteenth century, such as Dutch physician Johann Weyer's 1563 book, *De Praestigiis Daemonum* [The Deceptions of the Devil], purportedly debunked the widespread European belief in witchcraft that had led to the increasingly brutal prosecution of alleged witches, especially following the publication of Heinrich Kramer and Jacob Sprenger's witch-hunting manual, *The Malleus Maleficarum* in 1486.

More stable governments, more education, and more wealth enabled a greater number of people to turn their focus from merely surviving to thriving and coming up with ways to advance mankind. The Industrial Revolution, beginning in the late eighteenth century, saw the widespread use of machines and the rise of free-market capitalism. With a greater understanding of the world around them and a better quality of living, humanity began to squeeze God out of the public square. Even the United States, settled originally by English Separatists and Puritans, recognized the need for "separation of church and state" in its constitution. As human progress spread, justifications did too, and the enemy was behind them. The nineteenth century saw the abominable practice of slavery, a satanically influenced institution, come to a head in America. Its abolition both here and abroad was spearheaded by brave men and women of character, most of whom were followers of God; however, slavery's blight on our historical record still has residual consequences more than 150 years later. The enemy uses it even today to sow discord between the races.

The Twentieth Century: The Devil's Playground

The twentieth century saw a continued rise in both human progress and discord. The enemy found a foothold in both. Transportation and technology boomed with the proliferation of railways, automobiles, and airplanes. The dissemination of news and entertainment also blossomed with the advent of radio, film, television, and the internet. As these advancements spread, so did the enemy's nefarious application of them. The application of airplanes in war and the development of atomic weapons led to the most widespread destruction and death ever seen, in two devastating world wars, the second of which was aimed, once again, at exterminating the Jewish people. Totalitarian regimes, such as those in Nazi Germany and the Soviet Union, used new forms of mass media to spread propaganda about fascism and communism, respectively. America was not immune either, as it saw increasing discord due to major social and cultural changes, such as the Civil Rights Movement and the sexual revolution.

It was therefore fitting when in the 1997 film *The Devil's Advocate*, Al Pacino's character, the Devil himself, proclaimed, "Who, in their right mind, Kevin, could possibly deny the twentieth century was entirely mine? All of it, Kevin! All of it! Mine! I'm peaking, Kevin. It's my time now."[25]

The Approaching Final Battle and the Inevitable Victory of God

So far, the twenty-first century has been marked by rapid technological progress that has accelerated change in our culture so rapidly that it is disconcerting to many, leading to heightened stress and anxiety, the likes of which are reminiscent of the post–Industrial Revolution world. Technology promised to make us more efficient and productive, but it seems to have enslaved most of us. Staring at screens for hours a day has left many people feeling disconnected from others, anxious about life, and depressed.

This century has also seen other dramatic and rapid changes, such as climate concerns, racial tensions, increasing polarization in politics, the shift from tolerance to celebration of sexual perversion, the normalization of transgenderism, which was considered a mental disorder up until 2013, and ongoing geopolitical conflicts that have the world on the brink of nuclear war. The constant barrage of 24/7 news cycles promulgating mostly bad news or political discord has further polarized our society, as many label their political adversaries as morally reprehensible, even "deplorable."

None of this should be surprising. The history of the world is the history of a cosmic war. And the global and national circumstances will grow progressively worse before Jesus's promised return. Scriptures indicate that people will become increasingly selfish, boastful, proud, disobedient to their parents, slanderous, ungrateful, unloving, unforgiving, and even cruel. They will be reckless, having no self-control, haters of good, and lovers of money and pleasure rather than God.[26] But the good news is that there's a Hollywood ending to this story—the good guys win and the bad guys, after years of seemingly getting away with their crimes, get the justice they deserve.

God will have his way. After all, he is the author, producer, director, and star of this epic story we call history. You, too, have a role in this epic, because in this story, God has recorded every day of your life.[27] God decides how the last chapter ends, but you and I decide our role—either that of heroes living valiantly for some greater cause or of ineffectual bystanders passing time in our brief sojourn on earth.

5

LIFTING THE VEIL

Pay no attention to that man behind the curtain!

—ACTOR, FRANK MORGAN,
  AS THE WIZARD OF OZ

Introduction: The Hidden Battle Behind the Veil

We have established that there are unseen entities waging an unseen war, so it stands to reason that all of this occurs in an unseen location. As discussed in the previous chapter, one consequence of Satan's initial rebellion and mankind's subsequent Fall is that there is now a veil separating the visible, physical world from the invisible, spiritual one, where once there was not.

Veils generally have two purposes. The first can be for protection. When mankind sinned and fell in the Garden of Eden, the veil between the spiritual realm and the physical realm was placed in order to protect mankind from God's presence. Throughout the Bible, there are examples of men either hiding their faces or covering their faces for protection when in the presence of God, who is described in the Old and New Testaments as "a consuming fire."

The second obvious purpose of a veil is to conceal something, as the veil of a bride conceals her face until she is presented to her groom at the marriage altar, or as the curtain on a stage conceals the set and actors from the audience until the appropriate time. Satan and his demons use this purpose of the veil between the physical and spiritual realms to their advantage.

In guerrilla, ambush-style warfare, it is of the utmost importance to be stealthy and camouflaged. Modern, educated people in our Western society tend to be skeptical of phenomena they do not experience or for which there is seemingly no scientific proof. To many of them, all of life can be explained with science and psychology. The Devil and his comrades have done such a fine job of hiding behind the veil over the last 2,000 years, since Jesus made a public spectacle of them at his crucifixion, that many people today do not believe they exist at all.

But I sense the tide may be turning. As the pace of change in our society continues to escalate, as immoral and lascivious things become increasingly prominent and acceptable in our culture, and as the outright evil actions of men and women also increase, some are waking up to the idea that there simply must be some outside influence to make sense of it all. Why might these camouflaged enemies be manifesting now after centuries of hiding in the shadows?

The Role of Pagan gods in Human History

Powerful spirits, likely fallen angels, were once worshipped by the scattered nations as "gods," and ancient people from nations outside of Israel would often try to curry their favor by making sacrifices to them. These fallen elohim often required human blood sacrifice from their followers. These bloodthirsty, lesser gods would then grant their human followers, whom they despised, the desires of their hearts. Their leader, Satan, as god of this world, demonstrated this authority in the harsh Judean wilderness when he offered Jesus all the kingdoms of the world in return for Jesus's worship. At the time, the kingdoms of the world were in fact rightfully Satan's to give. But Jesus knew the bigger story that was unfolding.

Not heeding C. S. Lewis's warning against the bias of "chronological snobbery,"[1] many people today erroneously assert that people in ancient times believed in these lesser gods because they were simple-minded and superstitious and lacked scientific knowledge compared to modern people. I offer an alternative explanation: During the history after the Fall, before God became a man and entered our world, his Holy Spirit was only present for certain periods of time and for certain specific purposes. Because of this, the majority of the time, malevolent spirits could rule and reign openly and without a significant force in the world pushing back on them. Essentially, it was safe for them to manifest openly because they were at the top of the food chain and had no consistent rival restraining them. They relished appearing like gods to mortal man and openly rewarded their religious devotees who offered them worship. This is likely the reason that the first two commandments God gave to the Israelites after they were delivered from captivity in Egypt involved having no other gods besides him and an explicit prohibition against making, worshipping, and serving any image of a created thing.

Prior to Jesus's incarnation, every major civilization had a pantheon of gods who were not a figment of their primitive, superstitious imaginations but rather actual, created, and powerful spiritual beings who had rebelled against the one all-powerful creator, God. We see these pantheons not only in ancient civilizations, like those in Sumer and Babylonia, but also in more recent, sophisticated civilizations, such as Greece and Rome. People of these advanced civilizations did not believe that the idols and statues that they created were the gods themselves, as some people today suppose, but rather that the spirits needed a physical body to inhabit in order to live among them. An example of this can be seen in the Old Testament account of the Philistine god Dagon, recounted in the book of 1 Samuel Chapter 5.

The Philistines, it says, had captured the Ark of the Covenant from the Israelites, brought it to their chief god's temple in Ashdod, "and set it by Dagon."[2] It is interesting to note that the text reads "set it by Dagon," not "set it by Dagon's statue." Because the Ark of the Covenant housed the actual Spirit of God on earth, the Philistines were shocked to find the following morning that "Dagon was fallen upon his face to the earth, before the ark of the Lord."[3] They returned Dagon to his upright position; however, the following morning, they again found Dagon fallen, and this time, "the head of Dagon and both the palms of his hands were cut off."[4]

This is one of many examples in the Old Testament showing that the one true creator, God, is infinitely more powerful than any of the gods of the nations that were scattered after God confused their languages at the Tower of Babel. The Philistines were so convinced of the presence and power of Israel's God that they eventually returned the captured Ark of the Covenant to Israel.

The Defeat of the Fallen: Why the gods Went into Hiding

There were few monotheistic religions prior to Jesus's crucifixion, most prominent of which were the religion of the ancient Israelites, Zoroastrianism, and a brief failed trial of monotheism in Egypt by the pharaoh Akhenaten.[5] It is interesting to note that the polytheism that had dominated for thousands of years nearly disappeared from the world stage within a few centuries after the crucifixion, likely because the pantheon went into hiding following their resounding defeat. Pockets of polytheism did persist in India, the Far East, and in Indigenous tribes of Africa and the Americas, however.

After the crucifixion, God made good on his prophecy that he would send his Holy Spirit to permanently live within believers, giving them a new heart. The unclean spirits likely went out of humans as though it were a mass exorcism. God's Holy Spirit was to be continually present on earth from then on, being housed within the temple of each believer's body. Simultaneously, as the good news spread around the globe, the light of truth began to shine more brightly, driving the darkness into hiding.

The spirits that had once ruled entire nations, such as Egypt, had taken a mighty fall and now longed to return to the dwellings from which they had been banished. Now that human beings knew the truth, these malevolent spirit beings who were once considered gods could no longer blatantly and easily lie to humans. They receded into the background behind the veil, patiently working through devoted men and women to limit the spread of the gospel, undermine and minimize access to holy scriptures, and remove God himself from all aspects of public life. In essence, they have been in the process of emptying the culture of God, sweeping away any reference to absolute truth of scripture and putting in place a new social order that is upside down from what God intended. What is likely happening now is that these evil spirits are returning with other spirits more wicked than themselves, so that they may inhabit our land and dwell here, making the last state of our nation worse than the first. This possibility is given credence by the following statement Jesus made to his disciples:

When an unclean spirit goes out of a man, he goes through dry places, seeking rest, and finds none. Then he says, "I will return to my house from which I came." And when he comes, he finds it empty, swept, and put in order. Then he goes and takes with him seven other spirits more wicked than himself, and they enter and dwell there; and the last state of that man is worse than the first.[6]

Because the evil spirits were resoundingly defeated at the cross and subsequently disarmed, they simply had no choice but to go into hiding. Prior to that, there is no historical evidence that people were skeptical of their existence or their negative influence in the world. In fact, quite the opposite is true, and throughout the Bible, evil spirits were considered a reality, unlike today.

The Return of the Ancient Spirits

Having persuaded modern man that Satan does not even exist, Satan and his minions now seem to be growing bolder as they gain increasing cultural influence. In war, a soldier would not dare remove his camouflage unless the environment was safe to do so. Has our culture deteriorated morally to the point at which the spirits now feel safe to remove the camouflage and come out of hiding? At their core, these fallen angels have always wanted worship from mankind, and I believe they are now gradually emerging from behind the veil, thinking they will once again be revered as gods, as in ancient times.

Increasing paranormal manifestations, the proliferation of the subject in mass media entertainment (horror movies, sci-fi, and superheroes, for example), and the public's seemingly insatiable appetite for such are likely priming the pump for these evil spirits to utilize an end-times deception of some sort, a mass delusion that will be readily accepted due to our desensitization. Since they will not manifest and announce the truth that they are demonic, they will need a ruse as a cover story. Many believe they may present as aliens from a distant planet, who will claim they seeded humans long ago by combining their genetic material with primitive ape-like creatures. If so, they will likely dazzle with many lying signs and wonders. Perhaps they will claim to be benevolent and peaceful and attempt to convince us that God and his angels are the bad guys. This is all speculation, but we do know from Scripture that the most prominent feature of the end times will be deception, so we must remain vigilant and test the spirits.

Modern Pathways for Spiritual Deception

With the rise of experimental science, *empiricism* (the theory that all knowledge is derived from experience and observation) has gained prominence in our culture. People today often want to simply experience things for themselves before accepting them. They want to discover for themselves what, if anything, is behind the veil. These phenomena are called *occult*, because they are hidden and esoteric in nature. For example, there are retreats to offshore sights, in which people take hallucinogens, such as psilocybin, in a controlled environment for the express purpose of gaining insights from spiritual experiences while under the influence. Some travel to remote areas of Peru to try another culturally ritualistic hallucinogen, ayahuasca, for the same reasons. Others visit mediums, read tarot cards, play with Ouija boards, or follow horoscopes in hope of connecting with something spiritual that they are lacking in their own lives.

But the Bible states that actively seeking supernatural spiritual experiences is dangerous—so much so that God expressly forbids it. We were made for this earthly realm, and if we step onto the enemy's turf, we may get injured or worse. Think of the deleterious outcomes if we earth dwellers were to go diving in the ocean depths or travel to outer space without the proper gear, for example.

While it appears that ministering spirits, called *angels*, can come and go between the physical and spiritual realms at the behest of God, evil spirits are more constrained and must look for opportunities to enter our realm, what some call "open doors." Examples certainly include sin in general, but sexual sins, anger, bitterness, lying, trauma, and the taking of human life are particularly likely to attract and empower malevolent entities. Dabbling in occult practices and substance abuse are also common ways to widely open doors between the two worlds, which I have seen in my experience with patients. This is the reason that Timothy Leary in the 1960s influenced so many young hippies to seek spiritual enlightenment through hallucinogenic drugs, such as LSD. This, in turn, spawned psychedelic bands such as Jim Morrison's aptly named band, The Doors, who encouraged their fans to "break on through to the other side." The empty promises of the sex, drugs, and rock-and-roll lifestyle of the 1960s led to the "Jesus Revolution" of the early 1970s, in which thousands of young people, beginning in Southern California, were baptized and became followers of Jesus.

Occultism and sinful practices essentially grant evil spirits the right to enter through the opened doors and have access to and more direct influence in one's life. The foothold one unwittingly grants the Devil can soon become a stronghold—an impregnable citadel controlled by enemy forces. Therefore, I urge anyone who has opened such doors to hurry back to the other side to close them; I will discuss specifics of how to do so later in this book. While dramatic spiritual manifestations are rare, and demonic possession is even rarer, opening such doors does make them more likely. Since you can't "put the genie back in the bottle," so to speak, it is most prudent to heed God's warning and avoid opening such doors in the first place.

Scriptural Glimpses Behind the Veil

The only legitimate and safe way to explore what is behind the veil is to do so by examining the holy scriptures of religious faiths. There are numerous times in the Bible, for example, when God himself pulls back the curtain to give us a glimpse of the invisible spiritual realm that surrounds us. I will briefly describe four such instances in order to demonstrate several important truths we can learn about the unseen realm.

1. Daniel's Vision and the Battle of Angels

The first example is from the book of Daniel in the Old Testament. Some background: The nation of Israel was divided after the death of its third king, Solomon, into the ten northern tribes comprising the kingdom of Israel and two southern tribes called Judah. Judah was invaded and captured by the Babylonian Empire under King Nebuchadnezzar in 605 BC, sparking the first deportation of Jews to Babylon. The Babylonians took young Jewish men from noble families first, and the teenager Daniel was among these first deportees. He was given a new Babylonian name, Belteshazzar, and indoctrinated into the language, culture, and literature of the Babylonians. However, Daniel was determined not to defile himself by either eating food from the king's table or worshipping foreign gods, and the God of Israel gifted him with the ability to interpret the meaning of visions and dreams. Daniel so impressed King Nebuchadnezzar that he chose Daniel to enter the royal service. The king grew to trust Daniel's wisdom and judgment and eventually made him ruler over the whole province of Babylonia.

In the tenth chapter of the book of Daniel, after a three-week period of prayer and fasting, Daniel was standing on the bank of the Tigris River and saw a mighty angel appear in the sky. "His voice roared like a vast multitude of people," the Scripture says, and even though no one but Daniel could see the angel, the men with him were so terrified that they fled. Daniel, too, was afraid and fainted.[7]

Then, this mighty angel said, "Don't be afraid, Daniel. Since the first day you began to pray for understanding and to humble yourself before your God, your request has been heard in heaven. I have come in answer to your prayer. But for twenty-one days the spirit prince of the kingdom of Persia blocked my way. Then Michael, one of the archangels, came to help me, and I left him there with the spirit prince of the kingdom of Persia."[8]

Daniel's praying and fasting for his people had caught the attention not only of heaven but also of the powerful evil principality that governed the land of nearby Persia, which interfered with God's response. This fascinating glimpse into the unseen realm informs us of several truths about what goes on behind the veil.

First, it attests to the reality of the unseen battle going on in the spiritual realm, with active and intense fighting between holy and evil angels. Second, it shows that persistent prayer coupled with fasting is powerful and more likely to surpass evil spirits' attempts to hinder it, increasing the likelihood that it will be heard in heaven. Clearly, the fervent prayer of a righteous man accomplishes much, and God answers prayer that is in concert with his will. Third, this episode makes it clear that Satan and his forces try to hinder the work of good angels, who are ministering spirits dispatched by God himself. Some evil spirits, such as territorial principalities, are especially powerful. Even though the angel from heaven eventually broke free to accomplish his mission, he told Daniel: "Soon, I must return to fight against the spirit prince of the kingdom of Persia, and after that, the spirit prince of the kingdom of Greece will come."[9] The fight rages on behind the veil and will not cease until the King of kings returns in glory.

2. Elisha's Servant Sees the Heavenly Army

The next glimpse behind the veil occurred in the book of 2 Kings when the prophet Elisha and his servant were surrounded by the Aramean army, which was intent on harming them. The king of Aram had sent troops to Dothan to capture Elisha when he discovered that God had been revealing the king's secret battle plans to Elisha. When Elisha's servant awakened to find the city surrounded by an army with horses and chariots, he was understandably afraid.

In response to his fear, Elisha prayed for God to "open" his servant's eyes to see the reality of the spiritual army with chariots of fire filling the hills to defend Elisha and his servant. Clearly, the servant's physical ocular apparatus—made of rods, cones, a lens, and a retina—was functioning just fine. But God needed to temporarily lift the veil that normally concealed the spiritual world in order for the servant to believe that, to quote the book, "those who are with us are more than those who are with them."[10]

God can and does occasionally grant people the temporary ability to see into the spiritual realm to accomplish his purposes. In 2 Kings, God allowed his people to see his angel army in order to encourage them. And the 1975 book *Angels* by evangelist minister Billy Graham recounted an episode in which God allowed his enemies to see his angelic warriors behind the veil for a different reason—to terrify them.

Graham wrote about an instance John G. Paton had as a missionary to the New Hebrides Islands. One night, a group of armed natives surrounded Paton's hut. He was aware of this and prayed fervently for God's protection. Amazingly, the bloodthirsty mob left without harming Paton at all. Later, a converted native told Paton that the reason the natives did not attack his hut that fateful night was because they saw that his hut was guarded by large men in shining garments with drawn swords.[11]

The lessons here are that there is indeed a mighty unseen heavenly host of God's angels fighting on our behalf and that God can and occasionally will allow people to see behind the veil if it serves his purposes.

3. Job's Trial and the Divine Council

The third biblical example of the veil being lifted for our edification occurs in the book of Job, where we are permitted to view a meeting of the divine council in heaven, in which a host of angels are gathered. One of them is Satan, who appears to have been granted the powers of police patrol, prosecutor, and head of the penal system over human beings on earth.

"Where have you come from?" the Lord asked Satan.

Satan answered the Lord, "I have been patrolling the Earth, watching everything that's going on."

Then the Lord asked Satan, "Have you noticed my servant, Job? He is the finest man in all the Earth. He is blameless—a man of complete integrity. He fears God and stays away from evil."

Because Job had found favor in the eyes of God, Satan had an intense desire to see Job fall. So, Satan essentially acted as a crooked cop. Knowing that he had no evidence against Job, Satan resorted to a scheme of *entrapment*, defined legally as when a law enforcement agent acquires the evidence necessary to commence prosecution of a defendant by attempting to induce the defendant to engage in a criminal act that he would not otherwise have committed. In an act of arrogance and hubris that was typical of Satan, he told God that Job was righteous only because God had blessed him and put a hedge of protection around his life. God then granted Satan permission to test Job, not because Job had done anything wrong but rather because it was an opportunity to prove Job's faithfulness. The ruthless enemy, who is the god of this world, then orchestrated events culminating in Job losing most of his possessions, his business and livelihood, and even the lives of his precious children. Nevertheless, Job did not curse or even blame God, and Satan was defeated, left to wait for another opportunity.

That opportunity came at a future meeting of the divine council, in which God reminded Satan that Job had previously maintained his integrity, even though, God said, "You urged me to harm him without cause." Satan contended that if God took away Job's health, Job would then curse God. So, once again, God permitted Satan to afflict Job, this time with terrible boils from head to toe. Even though his own wife urged Job to "curse God and die," Job again proved his faithfulness by maintaining his integrity amid a trial of great adversity.

There are several important lessons to be gleaned from this account in the book of Job. In 1981, Rabbi Harold Kushner penned the bestseller *When Bad Things Happen to Good People.* My response to this title is, according to the full counsel of God, "They don't." That's not because bad things don't happen but because there are no good people, because all have sinned according to both the Old and New Testaments (Psalms and Romans, respectively).

One way God works to progressively conform sin-stained people into the image of his sinless son Jesus is by allowing trials to refine and test their faith by means of his permissive will. This in no way diminishes the sovereignty of God, because while God does, at times, allow satanic attacks to happen in order to test believers, Satan clearly must ask for and be granted permission to attack God's followers. Furthermore, God himself places limits on what Satan is permitted to do to his followers, as seen when God allowed Satan to rob Job of his health but not his life.

God is still in full control, and there is purpose behind the suffering, although the sufferer may never be privy to it. For example, although we, the readers, are given this behind-the-scenes glimpse of the divine council meeting and the reason for Job's suffering, Job himself never was during his lifetime.

4. The Rending of the Heavens at Jesus's Baptism

The final example of a biblical peek behind the veil occurred when God tore the veil at the baptism of Jesus by John the Baptist, marking the beginning of his public ministry. The Gospel of Mark uses the

Greek word *schizo* to describe the event, implying that God temporarily ripped open the veil in order to audibly express his pleasure with his only begotten Son, Jesus, and to confirm his anointing to the ministry. One important truth to be gleaned here is that all three persons of the Godhead were present simultaneously for this event, demonstrating the reality of the Trinity. Furthermore, the event was said to be a precursor to the day when, according to Jesus in the Gospel of Mark, the people "will see the Son of Man coming in clouds with great power and glory." The book of Revelation adds that every eye will see this event. The forecast is clear according to the Bible: God will one day soon permanently reopen the veil and send Jesus to come on the clouds, this time bringing judgment and establishing his eternal kingdom on earth.

The Coming Ultimate Revelation and Final Defeat of the Enemy

The Bible unequivocally states that the *apocalypse* is coming. Although this term has come to colloquially mean cataclysmic destruction, as purported to occur at the end of the world, the term is actually derived from the Greek word *apokalupsis*, a combination of two Greek words meaning "to remove a covering that hides something." Therefore, the final book of the Bible, The Apocalypse of St. John, or simply Revelation, provides the most extensive picture of what lies behind the veil. Its depictions of war in heaven, four supernatural horsemen, demons being freed from their prison in the bottomless pit and ascending to torment mankind, and the coming of a world ruler possessed by a powerful evil spirit called *Apollyon* are understandably difficult to comprehend. But to be forewarned is to be forearmed. Knowing that these evil spirits will one day return in full force from behind the veil will protect mankind from the coming deceptions.

The final and most important lesson we can take away from all these biblical glimpses behind the veil is that the good guys win, and God's plan will be accomplished despite apparent obstacles. Daniel's people were freed from exile in Babylon after seventy years and allowed to return to their promised land to rebuild Jerusalem. Good angels struggled with evil angels but still accomplished God's will. Elisha and his servant were not harmed by the Aramean army surrounding them; in fact, God answered Elisha's prayer to blind the soldiers, which enabled this one man to defeat an entire army. Job, though brutally attacked by Satan, stood firm in his faith and even worshipped God in the midst of his agony. And God worked through a lowly carpenter from the backwater province of Galilee to defeat Satan and his evil angels and to usher in salvation that is freely available to all of God's physical human family who will turn from their sins and believe.

Jesus is coming back at an appointed time that no man nor angel knows. Just as in *The Wizard of Oz* when Dorothy's beloved terrier, Toto, pulls back the curtain revealing that the supposed powerful, awe-inspiring wizard is merely an insecure man hiding behind the scenes, Jesus will one day pull back the curtain and stand in stark contrast to the inferior created being called Satan.

The prophet Isaiah described the scene when Satan is defeated once and for all: "Those who see you will gaze at you, they will consider you, saying, 'Is this the one who made the Earth tremble, who shook kingdoms, who made the world like a wilderness and overthrew its cities, who did not permit his prisoners to return home?'"[12]

One day soon, the veil will be lifted permanently, and Scripture says, "All that is secret will eventually be brought into the open, and everything that is concealed will be brought to light and made known to all."[13]

Section II

SPIRITUAL INTEL

6

TACTICAL INTEL: KNOW YOUR ENEMIES

If you know neither the enemy nor yourself,
you will succumb in every battle.

—SUN TZU, *THE ART OF WAR*

A key to victory in any war is knowledge, because "knowledge is power," as Francis Bacon famously asserted. Knowing your enemies, their appetites, and their tendencies is essential in warfare. This is called tactical intel.

Unfortunately, we do not face just one enemy in our fight. We face seven enemies—five of whom conspire together toward their sinister goals to steal, kill, and destroy. I will provide you a brief overview of each of our enemies as described by the Bible, but two enemies in particular—Satan and his demons—will be given their own chapters because of their critical importance.

Before we begin, remember that a wise and effective defense begins with knowledge.

Enemy #1: Yourself

Saint Augustine used to pray, "Lord, deliver me from that evil man, myself."[1] Walt Kelly once asserted, "We have met the enemy, and he is us."[2]

Both point to the same piece of wisdom: We should all take a look in the mirror before we look elsewhere for our enemies. Say hello to your surprising first enemy, the most intelligent and most dangerous animal on planet Earth: you.

Although the world system run by Satan tells us that mankind is essentially good, the Bible tells a different story: "All have turned aside; together they have become worthless; no one does good, not even one."[3]

As a human being, you were created with three parts: body, soul, and spirit.[4] The body is the part that enables you to interact with the physical world in which you live by means of your five physical senses, making you world-conscious. You have a body, but you are a living soul, the immaterial part that connects the physical and the spiritual realms.[5] The soul is your very essence, your unique personality, including your mind, will, and emotions, enabling you to be self-conscious.[6] The third and final component of your being is the spirit, that deepest part that enables you to contact God in the spiritual realm, beyond detection from our five senses, allowing you to be God-conscious.[7] While God formed other animated creatures containing a soul, mankind is his unique creation because we alone also possess a spirit. This is the most fundamental way in which mankind was created in God's image—God is a spiritual being.[8]

Tragically, your spirit was stillborn, because on that wonderful day of your birth, when your physical body housing your soul exited your mother's womb, one-third of your three-part nature was nonfunctional. It was born dead because of the sin nature you inherited from your ancestors when they rebelled against God thousands of years ago and fell from their sinless created state in the Garden of Eden.[9] Eve believed Satan when he told her the lie, "You shall not surely die," as a consequence of eating the forbidden fruit of the tree of the knowledge of good and evil. Eve's spirit, and then the spirit of all mankind following her, died at the moment of rebellion. That part of her being that enabled her to have unfettered communication and fellowship with God was gone. She and Adam were banished from the garden to toil on a now-cursed planet until the eventual day of their physical death.[10] To protect sinful mankind from a holy, sinless God, a veil between the spiritual and physical realms was put in place.

The environment God created to be ideally suited for all life, especially mankind, also became subject to degradation.[11] We see evidence of this in the second law of thermodynamics—entropy describes the increasing disorder within a system over the passage of time. The fall of God's entire created order best explains the progressively extreme climate change we now observe on our planet. Although we can and should be better stewards of the environment, the observable law of entropy and the testimony of the Bible suggest that the earth's ultimate decline is inevitable.[12] Sin and the gradual degradation of our ideally suited environment are the likely reasons that mankind's life expectancy has dropped from over 900 years at the time of Adam and Eve to approximately eighty years today.

Because your spirit was born dead, you are unknowingly born a slave into a kingdom of darkness led by the "prince of darkness," the term John Milton used for Satan in *Paradise Lost*. You are what the Bible calls a "natural" person, led to indulge the desires of your physical body. You are incapable of both receiving and understanding truth because your spirit is dead.[13] This is what the Bible means when it says that Satan works in the lives of unbelievers to blind their spiritual eyes and to snatch God's truth before it can potentially take root in one's heart.[14]

Lacking a spiritual filter, your soul (that is, your mind, will, and emotions) is heavily influenced by the world system under the control of the Devil and unclean spirits who have the legal right to enter the house of your soul and fill the void where your spirit would reside if it were not dead. You seek neither God nor spiritual things because you lack the capacity and are too busy indulging your fleshly appetites and being unduly influenced by the "great evil princes of darkness who rule this world."[15] The things of God are utter foolishness to you.[16] You have become your own enemy because you are unwittingly destined to be a casualty in the unseen war, having the same ultimate fate of eternal punishment as that of Satan and his demon horde.

With all of this working against you, what hope of escape could you possibly have from being enslaved to sin and bodily appetites in this kingdom of darkness? You might seem like a good person compared to your neighbor but not when compared to the standard of a perfect, sinless God. There is no number of good deeds that will cancel out your sin. You need help. You need someone to save you from this hopeless enslavement into which you were born. Deliverance and freedom are indeed possible, but from a very unlikely source—your second enemy.

Enemy #2: God

God created mankind, his physical family, to be his image-bearers, who would carry out his will on earth. But when mankind made the decision to disobey God by believing Satan's lies and eating the forbidden fruit, sin entered our hearts and the entire created world, making us enemies of God.[17] Our ancestors essentially declared citizenship to the kingdom of darkness and its god.[18] They understandably became afraid of God the Creator's wrath and judgment and immediately attempted to hide from him.

God, in turn, banished them from his presence, because he is holy and cannot look upon sin. God had warned them that they would die if they rebelled, but Adam and Eve chose to believe Satan's lie that they would not die but instead become gods themselves.[19]

Contrary to God's original intention, mankind's spirit immediately died, and our bodies immediately became subject to sickness, decay, and eventual death. Mankind became friendly toward and comfortable with the world system that Satan was building. This friendship with the world further solidified mankind's enmity toward God.[20]

The difference between enemy #2 and enemy #1 is that you cannot overcome enemy #2. He is too powerful—all-powerful, in fact. Since fighting this enemy is not a viable option, the only remaining alternative is to surrender in the hope of brokering a favorable peace treaty.

Every natural, spirit-dead person returns evil for evil, but this enemy is unique in all the universe. He returns good for evil, and his unique kind of love—called *agape* in Greek—is sacrificial, serving, and full of unmerited grace and mercy. Although you are against God, he is surprisingly not against you. The startling reality is that God is for you and wants to make peace.[21]

Although you lack the capacity and desire to seek God with your whole body, mind, and heart, your second enemy is not only willing to come to peace terms with you but also even initiates the process of reconciliation.[22] However, the only way God can reconcile with humans is to restore us to our original, sinless, created state. So, how does God accomplish this restoration? By means of salvation.[23] In fact, the very name of Jesus, whom he sent to be a substitutionary sacrifice, means "Yahweh is salvation."[24] God's salvation plan has three parts, each addressing a component of our tripartite nature.

In the first stage of salvation, God deals with your spirit by saving you from the penalty of your sin. Most natural persons only come to their senses and hear God calling for them when they find that the promises of the world and the flesh have left them empty and unfulfilled, which often occurs when they face a crisis in their lives that they are unable to fix themselves. The outcome often relies upon how one responds to adversity. Hence, despite what our culture might tell us, not all adversity in life is bad, especially when it points you to God. If you wisely decide to accept your second enemy's peace terms, you simultaneously overcome your first enemy, yourself. It is only when you accept God's peace terms through Jesus's sacrifice that you are instantaneously returned to good standing with God, a term called *justification*. And it is only when you have overcome yourself and entered peace with God that you will be able to effectively fight the other five enemies gunning for you. Fortunately, God sends his life-giving Spirit to those restored to him in order to empower them to fight and win the spiritual battles they will face for the rest of their lives on earth. Once you have chosen sides and transferred your citizenship from the kingdom of darkness to the Kingdom of Light, God equips you with armor for protection and weapons to successfully wage war against your spiritual foes.[25]

The second phase of salvation refers specifically to the second component of our tripartite nature, the soul, which is our mind, will, and emotions. This lifelong process is termed *sanctification*, and it refers to our gradual transformation into the likeness of Christ's nature.[26] Sanctification saves us from the power of sin and is accomplished by the Holy Spirit continually renewing our mind and giving us both the desire and the power to carry out God's will on earth.[27] Scripture says we can track our progress and know exactly where we are on the road to sanctification by gauging the degree to which we are manifesting the fruits of the Spirit—"love, joy, peace, patience, kindness, goodness, gentleness, and self-control."[28] Constantly connecting with God and carrying out his desires for the world progressively conforms us to his image and brings out this fruit of the Spirit in our lives. This is why Jesus told Satan, "Man must not live on bread alone but by every word that proceeds out of the mouth of God."[29]

The final and future phase of salvation pertains to the physical body and is the promise called *glorification*, in which we are saved from the very presence of sin itself. Glorification refers to the instantaneous shedding of our old physical body with its sin nature for a new, glorified body incapable of sin, sickness, decay, or death. This new body will be an eternal one fit to live forever on a new earth with God and other redeemed souls. It is of vital importance that we put on the "Helmet of Salvation" that God has provided us for our protection and fully realize that although God may not heal all our physical infirmities, injuries, and deformities during our brief lives on earth, for reasons we cannot comprehend, he will do so eventually.[30] This ultimate redemption of our bodies at Jesus's triumphal return is our blessed hope, our rock-solid assurance of God's love for us, and his desire to fully restore what mankind wrecked by means of our rebellion.[31]

To sum it up, your second enemy will become your all-powerful ally when you agree to his gracious terms of peace. If you accept this free gift of salvation, God will cancel the death penalty assigned to you for your treasonous rebellion. Additionally, he promises to gradually change your nature into the likeness of his, eventually restoring you to your intended state at creation. And finally, God promises to reward you with a new glorified body, impervious to death, pain, sickness, or injury so that you can live with him on a new earth free from sin, demons, and the Devil. When God is your ally, you are saved from the penalty of sin and armed to defeat the power of sin in your own life. God promises that he will eventually rid the earth of your next five enemies and provides a plan to overcome their attacks until that happens.

Enemy #3: The Flesh

When you accept Christ's substitutionary, sacrificial death on the cross as payment for your sins, God initiates his plan of salvation, but your inherited sin nature unfortunately remains until he redeems your physical body someday in the future. Thus, what the Bible calls "the flesh" persists and is the weak link that Satan and his demons primarily use to tempt us to continue to sin, despite having a reborn spirit.[32]

Satan prefers to have us live on a lower plane, like animals, where we are slaves to our desires and appetites. As we will see later, he often sends fiery darts to enflame the passions of our flesh, tempting us to sin.[33] The flesh is the natural fallen part of you that is subject to your body's appetites, making you an unwitting slave to the world system. The flesh was technically not your enemy until you were given a new spirit by God. At that moment, this traitor within you, who works in concert with the demons, essentially declared civil war.[34] The fleshly part of your body fights against your God-given spirit.

There is only one way to defeat this enemy: Kill it.[35] You can do this in two ways, which are ultimately one and the same: 1) symbolically "crucify" your enemy every day, willingly denying your sinful temptations[36] or 2) starve your enemy by neglecting its sinful desires so regularly that it loses its appeal.[37]

Unfortunately, both crucifixion and starvation are slow and excruciatingly painful ways to die. Crucifixion could take up to four days to claim its victim's life, and starvation typically takes between several weeks and several months. Not surprisingly, the flesh puts up intense resistance to these slow, horrific means of death. The Greek verb used in Galatians 5:24, translated as "have crucified," is in the active voice and hints that the believer must continually, metaphorically nail the flesh to the cross. The flesh essentially remains alive, constantly fighting to break free from the cross, but because it is bound, it is unable to act on its desires. But note carefully that the desires of your fleshly appetites remain. This slow death is part of the salvation process called sanctification, which was discussed earlier. The flesh will only die once you are given a redeemed, glorified body, free of a sin nature. Until then, your enemy called the flesh should grow increasingly weaker as the sanctification process saves you from the power of sin.

It is important that we do not repeatedly yield to the desires of the flesh, because this gives the Devil a foothold in our lives that can be progressively built into a stronghold.[38] The vital issue is not simply that we have God's Holy Spirit in us but that we submit to his leading, because he alone possesses the power to defeat our flesh.

Enemy #4: The World

"If we find ourselves with a desire that nothing in this world can satisfy," noted C. S. Lewis, "the most probable explanation is that we were made for another world."[39] The Apostle John took this further when he wrote to followers of Jesus, "Do not love the world or anything in the world."[40] That's right, the God of love actually hates certain things, and he commands us to follow suit in order to protect us.

You might be wondering: *Why should we not love this world and all the perks, pleasures, and entertainment it has to offer?* The answer might be simpler than you realize. We should not love the world because, believe it or not, the world hates you and is under the control of the Devil himself.

According to the Bible, everything God had created before the Fall of mankind was "good."[41] The redefining of good and evil that goes on to this very day at an alarmingly accelerating pace began in the Garden of Eden when Satan questioned Eve about God's love, his word, and his motives.[42] When mankind was stripped of our authority over the earth due to our original sin, Satan assumed control and became the god of this world.[43] Satan then developed and governed an intricate system, designed to draw mankind away using what God called "the lust of the flesh, the lust of the eyes, and the pride of life."[44] It is a system in total rebellion against God that turns the world upside down by labeling what is good *evil* and what is evil *good*.

This world system is an intricate network that has its far-reaching tentacles in nearly every facet of human life, including government, education, religion, business, healthcare, arts, science, literature, philosophy, sports, media, and entertainment, to name a few. It promotes wrong priorities and chasing treasures on earth, like fame, fortune, and accolades. While most people are unwitting slaves to this system, following their instincts as an animal would, I believe that Satan also actively patrols the earth looking for capable and willing men and women he can entice with fame and fortune to serve in his kingdom. He likewise takes note of his especially capable and blessed enemies serving God's kingdom and looks to neutralize them with discouragement, disasters, disease, and loss, as in the case of Job in the Old Testament.[45]

I have heard this world system called "your friendly enemy," because by gratifying the natural desires of our flesh, it entices us to follow a path of least resistance that, unbeknownst to us, leads to enmity toward God and eventual destruction.[46] We are like sheep without a shepherd, easily led to the slaughter.[47] These natural appetites are not bad in and of themselves but must be controlled and satisfied in the proper timing and context that God intended. An example is our sexual appetite, which is normal and good to solidify a biblically defined marital relationship as one flesh and to bring about procreation in that context. However, the world system turns this definition of a natural, God-given appetite upside down by encouraging us to gratify sexual desires at the wrong time and in the improper context.

This enticing world system designed to draw us away from God, and thus unwittingly into danger, reminds me of the medieval German folktale—believed to have some basis in fact—called the Pied Piper of Hamelin. The story recounts that a piper was hired to rid the village of a rat infestation, but after he successfully did so, the townspeople refused to pay him his wages as promised. So, he sought revenge by donning a multicolored outfit and playing a sweet melody on his flute that served to draw the children of Hamelin to follow him out of town, never to be seen again. The evidence for this tale being an anecdote rather than allegory stems from the fact that there is still today a plaque in the tiny hamlet that reads:

In the year 1284 on the day of [Saints] John and Paul, June 26, 130 children born in Hamelin were lured by a piper clothed in many colors to Calvary near the Koppen [and] lost.[48]

Similar to the Pied Piper, Satan is a vindictive enemy with designs to lure us away from our Creator with numerous worldly enticements that are pleasant and seemingly harmless but ultimately lead us to our demise. All of mankind being born into this system, and hence, knowing no other way of doing, having, or being, reminds me of Aristotle's question, "Does a fish know that it is wet?"

The answer is, "Not until it is taken out of the water."

Exposure to an unnatural and inherently uncomfortable environment makes the fish long for its former security and comfort in the water. This is essentially what happens when we natural citizens are exposed to devout, God-worshipping strangers. We find these "foreigners" from the kingdom of God who are living in our land to be odd in their beliefs, interests, desires, habits, dress, music, and morality.[49] As natural-born citizens of the kingdom of the world, we erroneously believe that mankind should be free because people are basically good. And being good people ourselves, we are therefore willing to tolerate these foreigners, as long as they do not infringe upon our freedoms and rights or try to push their beliefs upon us.

But like the fish, we only discover that we are living in a dark world when we are exposed to the light these devout foreigners possess by their very nature. When these foreigners are lukewarm and carrying a dim light, we give them little thought, but when they are devout and assertive about their beliefs, it chafes against us and pushes the limits of our tolerance. Once citizens of this foreign Kingdom of Light make us uncomfortable by exposing the darkness and seemingly infringe upon our freedoms, the world system springs into action to suppress or altogether eliminate them because they are an existential threat to our very way of life.

There are two very different kingdoms at odds with each other: the kingdom of the world run by Satan and the kingdom of God. The invisible enemy, Satan, is the force behind the visible enemy at war with God's people—the culture. Humans are de facto citizens of this world system until they renounce their citizenship at some point and declare allegiance to God, at which time they are granted citizenship to his kingdom.[50] Three things occur when you change your citizenship: You go from 1) being in the world to being transferred to heavenly places, 2) following Satan, the prince of the power of the air, to following the Prince of Peace, and 3) being dead from following your sinful nature to being alive because of your renewed spirit.[51]

But the change of citizenship comes with a cost. Jesus told his disciples that once anyone becomes a citizen in God's kingdom, he or she would have tribulation in this world.[52] In other words, you will still live in this world, but you are no longer to be conformed to it or love it.[53] As a result, the world will hate you without cause, just as it hated Jesus.[54] You are now living with a bull's-eye on your back in hostile enemy territory. So how can you defeat your formidable foe?

The answer lies in the fact that once you surrender to God and renounce your citizenship in the world, the omnipotent, omnipresent King of the Universe comes to live within you, reviving your dead spirit. This is the reason Scripture states, "He who is in you is greater than he who is in the world."[55] God is not equal and opposite of Satan. God created Satan, and, by definition, the Creator is greater than the creation. The ultimate victory is with God's camp. How do we know we're in the right camp?

Faith.

The Shield of Faith is your defensive weapon. Scripture says, "with which you can extinguish all the fiery darts of the evil one," the arrows Satan shoots at you to enflame your natural passions for "the lust of the flesh, the lust of the eyes, and the pride of life."[56]

Enemy #5: The Devil

This anointed cherub was perhaps God's greatest created being before his rebellion, at which time he became *ha-satan*, "the adversary," who essentially declared war with God. Unable to get to God directly, the Devil instead goes after God's beloved children, created in his image. Mankind is thus a pawn in the fight against this formidable enemy who does not fight fair. Satan is older and smarter, possesses supernatural powers, controls the entire world system, wears disguises or cannot be seen, and has plausible lies, a vast army with a battle plan, a propaganda machine, and the ability to injure us before we even know we are in a fight. This prince of the power of the air and god of this world will be discussed further in Chapter 7.

Enemy #6: Demons

Innumerable malevolent spiritual beings called "unclean spirits" are part of Satan's vast army, which has a clear hierarchy, like a human national military. Like humans, they have unique personalities and varying degrees of abilities. Lower-level demons are essentially opportunistic spiritual parasites that feed on our emotions and try to influence humans to have evil thoughts or perform evil acts, whereas higher-ranking demons likely have greater power and authority—even being in charge of entire nations. These sinister foes will be discussed in greater depth in Chapter 8.

Enemy #7: The Children of Disobedience

We have established that God has adopted human children, but Satan also has children, according to Scripture.[57] The Apostle Paul uses the title "the children of disobedience" three times to refer to unbelievers under the control of Satan's spirit.[58] While God disciplines and corrects his own children, whom he loves, Satan's "children of disobedience" are often rewarded by their diabolical father with pleasure, possessions, and status but are ultimately destined to face God's wrath if they do not change sides.[59]

Although some human children of the Devil are passively and unknowingly used by Satan to help run the various branches of the world system or to persecute believers, others are willing participants, who very intentionally agree to do the Devil's bidding. We should not be dismissive of accounts of people allegedly selling their souls to the Devil. Pastor Joe Schimmel of Good Fight Ministries created an in-depth, ten-hour video series titled *They Sold Their Souls for Rock 'n' Roll*, which chronicles numerous musical artists, many of whom admit in their own words to making a bargain with dark forces or using unseen spiritual powers to enable them to both write and perform their popular music.

Since the Devil is neither omnipresent nor omniscient like God himself, I believe it is likely that Satan patrols the earth, searching for capable, talented, and gifted humans whom he can entice with wealth and positions of power and prominence to join his family.[60] After all, Scripture states that he attempted to use these very same schemes to tempt Jesus in the Judaean desert, offering him all the kingdoms of the world and subsequent authority over them in exchange for worshipping Satan.[61]

These sons of disobedience are Satan's frontline human foot soldiers, expendable pawns in the war against God, who are discarded by their ruthless adoptive father once their usefulness to him has run its course. Like Esau in the Old Testament, they are willing to relinquish their birthright, inheritance, and eternal treasures in heaven for temporal earthly comforts and possessions offered by their diabolical adoptive father, only to later realize that these do not satisfy in the long run nor stand the test of time.[62] These sons of disobedience are used to doing Satan's dirty work of spreading poison to the masses by means of the culture and the world system to accomplish his sinister goals to steal, kill, and destroy anything linked to God's kingdom.

Believers are called to resist the "children of disobedience" we face in the world by seeking to repay their evil not with vengeance but with good.[63] It is important to realize that these final enemies could still be turned into allies and transferred from the kingdom of darkness to the Kingdom of Light. The real enemies are the invisible sinister forces behind the visible human persecutors and purveyors of filth. People come and go, but the demonic spirits behind them remain, and so it is essential for us to grasp that, as Scripture states, "We are not fighting against flesh-and-blood enemies, but against evil rulers and authorities of the unseen world, against mighty powers in this dark world, and against evil spirits in the heavenly places."[64]

These are our seven enemies in this invisible cosmic war. But before we turn the page on this topic, we need to turn our attention to a more thorough investigation of the powerful mastermind behind it all, Satan himself.

7

THE GOD OF THIS WORLD

My dear brethren, never forget, when you hear the progress of wisdom vaunted, that the cleverest ruse of the Devil is to persuade you he does not exist!

—CHARLES BAUDELAIRE

The ultimate villain of history is indeed real and quite powerful. But his primary character trait is deceitfulness. How else could he so overwhelmingly convince modern man that he is neither real nor powerful?

Although the tide may be starting to turn as people seem to be awakening from their spiritual slumber, most people, including many Christians, still do not believe the Devil exists. And for those open to his existence, Satan has run quite an effective propaganda campaign suggesting that he is merely a trickster if he exists at all—a joke in tight red underwear and a goatee who pokes unsuspecting folks with his pitchfork when they bend over.

God is good and, according to the first book of the Jewish Pentateuch, everything he created was also good. It is hypothesized that one of the main reasons for creation is that God desired to have a family, so he created both spiritual and physical beings to be his image-bearers in their respective realms that initially overlapped with each other.

The Creator is, by definition, greater than anything in his creation.[1] Contrary to what many assume, God did not create evil, nor did he create a devil. In fact, he created a beautiful, vastly talented, and gifted "anointed cherub" named Lucifer who, because of his great pride, rebelled against God. Desiring to become like the Most High, Satan essentially declared war on God and both his spiritual and physical children.[2]

This cosmic spiritual battle is not dualistic in nature, in which two equal but opposite forces of good and evil are locked in a fierce struggle to determine the ultimate fate of the universe. Since God is omnipotent and above his created beings, including the powerful rebellious cherub, the ultimate outcome of the war is not in question.

This leads to the question of why God doesn't just end all this suffering and return in triumph, defeating the evil forces that war against him and his beloved created human and spiritual families once and for all.

Many theologians believe it is because God does not want any of his beloved human imagers to perish. In other words, he is mercifully patient, allowing people time to turn back to him willingly.[3] This is the reason that God's rescue plan has two phases, according to the Christian faith.

Phase one occurred when God's Messiah veiled his glory in human flesh and came to earth to live among mankind for one purpose: to offer himself as a perfect, sinless sacrifice for the past, present, and future sins of all mankind.

Phase two of the rescue plan is a future event when the Messiah will return to earth to cast out its current ruler, judge the wicked, and take his rightful place as King of kings.

Since the Devil is very powerful but not all-powerful, like his Creator, he cannot possibly defeat God. So, what is his reason for fighting a war he cannot possibly win?

As a doctor trained to understand the mind and its motives behind behavior, I have some thoughts that are, admittedly, purely speculative. The first possible reason could be because he simply has no other choice but to fight onward, because surrender means judgment and certain eternal death. Essentially, Satan made a tragically bad decision and started down a road from which he cannot turn back, so now he is in perpetual fight-or-flight mode. Most of us have probably seen that even when the most docile animal gets backed into a corner, it becomes quite aggressive, even ferocious, because it has no options and is in mortal danger.

I believe a second possible explanation is that Satan's narcissistic rage over time has progressed into a delusional mindset to the point where he erroneously thinks he can actually win this war. Possible evidence for this is that as time draws us closer to the Messiah's return, things in the world's governments and cultures have increasingly become so bizarre that many of the circumstances today simply do not make rational sense and seem to be driven by fixed false beliefs that we would label delusions in a clinical setting.

If my first two theories are not correct, I believe a final possible explanation is that this brilliant, evil prosecutor clings to the hope that he might win on a legal technicality by finding some loophole the Judge will have no choice but to honor.

Whatever the real reason, we know that Satan hates God's human children and is literally hell-bent on taking as many of God's imagers with him into perdition as he can. The good news is that, unlike the fallen angels and their leader, we humans have an opportunity to be healed of our spiritual blindness and come to our senses. Humans should learn from Lucifer's tragic story: We cannot fight God, so it is wisest to submit to him while we still have time.

The Enemy's Many Names

In the Old Testament, names were extremely important, often conveying some fundamental character trait about the individual. So, examining the names of mankind's ultimate adversary will give you a richer and more historically grounded understanding of this fallen, anointed cherub, which may be of benefit in the battle against illness.

Satan

In the Old Testament, nearly all references to the being called Satan are actually *ha-satan* in the Hebrew language. In Hebrew, *ha* is the definite article *the*. This means that the term *ha-satan* initially referred not to a proper name but to a title or office, translated as "the adversary" or "the accuser." In Hebrew, as in English, proper names do not have *the* attached to them (hence, I am not *the Tom*). In Old Testament Hebrew, the word *satan* is often used in a general way, as a noun twenty-seven times and as a verb six times. Thus, in Hebrew, the noun and verb can have the nontechnical meaning of *standing opposed to someone as an adversary*. It is used to describe both human terrestrial opponents and supernatural celestial opponents in the Old Testament.

Old Testament scholar Michael Heiser, PhD, proposed that Satan was originally part of God's divine council, a group of spiritual beings who serve as God's administrators.[4] Heiser's belief was that Satan was tasked with the role of testing and accusing humans and that the rebellion of some divine beings, including Satan, is part of a broader narrative of cosmic conflict, with Satan's fall being a pivotal event that led to his adversarial role.

Adversary

God created Lucifer as the highest-ranking angel of his spiritual family, the "anointed cherub" who was the epitome of beauty, wisdom, and splendor.[5] Aside from God himself, Lucifer was the most glorious being imaginable, the pinnacle of all created beings. He, along with all of the angels, is said to have praised God and "shouted for joy" at the laying of the foundation of the earth, probably on day two or three of creation.[6]

However, the first narcissist was born when Lucifer later realized that he was required by God to serve the first human, Adam, who was made from dust and who was destined to become positionally greater than he. Lucifer's pride likely swelled, and he became angry at God. Lucifer functioned well as long as his beauty, wisdom, and splendor were recognized and mirrored back to him, but God commanding him to be a servant to a lower life form created from dirt was simply intolerable. He felt his gifts entitled him to lead, not to serve, and so in his pride he decided to lead a coup. The prophet Isaiah records God recounting Lucifer's resolutions in the face of his narcissistic collapse:

> For you said to yourself, "I will ascend to heaven and set my throne above God's stars [the other angelic beings]. I will preside on the mountain of the gods far away in the north. I will climb to the highest heavens and be like the Most High."[7]

At that point of rebellion, Lucifer, the beautiful and gifted angel, became *ha-satan* in Hebrew, meaning "the adversary," a term that encapsulates his role as an opponent of both God and humanity. The Devil and God are not equal and opposite. Since Satan knew he could not defeat the omnipotent God by taking him on directly, he searched for legal loopholes and planned an indirect route of attack.

Satan likely believed he could eliminate his human rivals and hurt God most by enticing humans to sin, thereby forcing God to render justice by imposing the death penalty against his own beloved children. This plan seemed to work, initially, as Satan took the title deed to the earth, to which mankind had lost legal right, and then exalted himself as the god of his seized domain.[8] However, Satan was likely crestfallen to learn that God, in his divine foreknowledge, had secretly formulated a plan before creation ever took place to send a redeemer who would rescue mankind from the death penalty they deserved. Since mankind would not die immediately, as Satan had supposed, he decided that humans must be controlled, and the best way to do that was by blinding them to spiritual realities and enslaving them in the physical realm.

By the time of the New Testament writing, the adversary's exploits over thousands of years had earned him the proper nickname of Satan, because he had become the very epitome of adversary. In fact, the New Testament writings emphasize Satan's adversarial nature. For instance, the Apostle Peter describes him as a "roaring lion" seeking to devour, while the Apostle Paul speaks of the spiritual struggle against the "powers of this dark world."[9]

The designation of Satan as an adversary underscores the reality of spiritual warfare and the need for people fighting illness to be vigilant and to resist the Devil's schemes through faith, prayer, and understanding of the spiritual truths outlined in holy scripture.

As the adversary, Satan represents ongoing opposition to God's divine order and purposes. This manifests in various forms, including deception, temptation, and direct confrontation. He embodies the forces that seek to disrupt, corrupt, and destroy the good that God has created, and in his adversarial role, Satan has rightly become the very personification of evil today.

Accuser

In the Old Testament, the term *ha-satan* can also mean "the accuser." This term encapsulates the Devil's function in the divine courtroom, where he is likened to a passionate prosecuting attorney who goes strictly by the book in bringing charges against humanity before God. In both the Old Testament books of Job and Zechariah, ha-satan appears as a member of the divine council, performing this role of a prosecutor under God's sovereignty.

First, there is the case of Job, a very righteous and materially blessed man who likely lived in the Middle East more than 4,000 years ago. Ha-satan acts as an accuser before God, challenging Job's righteousness. God then grants the accuser the authority to test the faith and integrity of Job, but it is vitally important to realize that God is sovereign and puts limits on Satan, who cannot act in any way toward Job without legal right or permission from God.[10]

A second Old Testament example of Satan acting as a prosecutor involves a vision from the prophet Zechariah, who sees Satan stand as an accuser against Joshua, the high priest, highlighting his role in opposing God's chosen representatives and their mission.[11] The righteous and just Judge responds by rebuking Satan, emphasizing God's sovereignty over the accuser's charges.

In the New Testament, Satan is also seen as a prosecutor, who is called "the accuser of the brethren" in the book of Revelation.[12] Satan is said to accuse believers before God "day and night," highlighting the continuous and relentless nature of the prosecutor's accusations. This relentless adversarial stance is a core aspect of his character.

Satan's role in seeking to highlight human shortcomings and demand our condemnation is contrasted with Christ's role as an advocate, in which he personally intercedes on behalf of believers, offering forgiveness and redemption.[13] The Apostle Paul states that once we accept this forgiveness and redemption, "there is no condemnation for those who belong to Christ Jesus."[14]

Recognizing the Devil as an accuser is crucial for understanding the nature of spiritual warfare. The word *devil* means "slanderer," one who makes false statements damaging to a person's reputation. So, not only does Satan accuse others, but he falsely accuses them, due to the lying nature of his character. Even though the adversary's railing accusations do not stick to believers, his claims can still lead us to feelings of guilt, shame, and unworthiness. Hence, some feelings of guilt and shame that we experience may be seen as manifestations of the Devil's accusations, emphasizing the need for spiritual interventions, such as the 12 Steps of Ruachiatry we will unpack later.

To be optimally successful and fight against illness, we must be equipped to counteract accusations with the truth of our identity in God and the assurance of God's forgiveness. As patients in search of healing, learning to expect accusations as part of spiritual opposition emboldens us to stand firm in our faith and grow in perseverance.

An interesting side note, albeit a non-scriptural one, is that perhaps the Devil is not only a prosecutor accusing the righteous but also a defense attorney for the wicked, as depicted in the motion picture *The Devil's Advocate*, starring Al Pacino and Keanu Reeves. While this is clearly pure speculation, it may help us understand why so many wicked lawbreakers seemingly escape justice for their transgressions during their lives on earth. After all, the Devil does have adopted human offspring called "the children of disobedience," who do his will in opposition to God.[15] So, would we not expect a corrupt prosecutor to either decline to bring charges against his own children or defend them vigorously so that they can remain free to do his bidding?

Murderer

The motive for the Devil's crimes is clear: wounded pride followed by narcissistic rage followed closely by covetousness and vengeance. Perhaps the Devil's anger was due to God's requirement that he humble himself and serve the first human, whom Satan viewed as his inferior rival. The Apostle Paul stated that there is a foreseeable progression of anger about which we must be knowledgeable in order to control it. He instructed the first-century Ephesian church to "Let all bitterness, wrath, anger, clamor, and evil speaking be put away from you, with all malice."[16] The culmination of unmanaged anger is malice or, in Satan's case, the evil intention to murder God's human imagers.

Jesus taught that the unmanaged emotion of anger is the precursor to the act of murder when he told his disciples that not only are you guilty if you violate the sixth commandment to not kill but also that "if you are even angry with someone, you are subject to judgment!"[17] Legally, malice is the mens rea, or criminal intent, that is required for the crime of murder.

Although the Devil is not directly referred to as a murderer in the book of Genesis, his role in the Fall of humanity through deception and temptation by the "serpent" led to spiritual and eventual physical death. His motive of murder was accomplished by his method of deception, which initiated the process of sin and death entering the world, making him the ultimate source of mortality. Jesus rightly called the Devil "a murderer from the beginning" and "the father of lies," statements suggesting that Satan's role as the original bringer of death indeed began with his deceit and corruption of truth.[18] Satan thus embodies the ultimate opposition to life, in stark contrast with God's nature as the giver and sustainer of life.

Scripture further insinuates that all subsequent murderers of God's human imagers, beginning with Cain killing his brother,

Abel, have been unduly influenced by the evil one.[19] Since it is widely considered a scientific fact that humans have an instinctual drive to procreate and pass on their genes, it stands to reason that whenever we observe humans trying to kill other humans (be it through suicide, murder, abortion, or war), it is unnatural in that it goes against biological drives to continue the species. Many today choose to believe that unnatural acts such as suicide and murder, for example, are the product of a psychologically or biochemically disordered mind, and in some cases, those factors are indeed either causative or strongly contributory. However, when a natural explanation is lacking, in some cases, I believe the situation warrants consideration of a supernatural cause—an evil, spiritual force driving the desire and subsequent behavior.

Liar

Leonard Ravenhill said, "The Devil has two major tricks with people. One is, 'You're so good you don't need to be saved.' The other is, 'You're so bad you can't be saved.' And he's a liar on both counts."[20]

Among the various names attributed to the Devil in biblical literature, *liar* stands out as a significant descriptor of both his character and actions. This designation highlights the fundamental opposition between truth, as represented by God, and falsehood, as embodied by the Devil. Jesus described the Devil as "a liar."[21] This original liar, from whom all falsehoods ultimately originate, introduced sin into the human experience by deceiving Eve with a mixture of half-truths and blatant falsehoods. If his motives are vengeance and covetousness fueled by a narcissistic wound, and his crime is murder, then his method is deception. His kingdom of darkness is built and maintained on a foundation of lies, and his role encompasses both overt deceptions and subtler forms of misleading. For example, the Apostle Paul warned the first-century Corinthian church that Satan disguises himself as an "angel of light," indicating his capacity for deception and the danger of his lies.[22]

By labeling the Devil a liar, the Bible underscores the nature of deceit as inherently evil. Lies distort reality, undermine trust, and lead individuals away from God's truth. The Devil's lies are fundamentally opposed to the very nature of God, who is often referred to as truth itself.[23] The modern proliferation of misinformation, "fake news," and deceit that increasingly undermine public trust and destabilize society can be viewed as a modern manifestation of Satan's deceptive tactics, making the biblical depiction of the Devil as a liar all the more relevant today.

Recognizing the Devil as a liar reinforces the need for us humans to exercise vigilance, discernment, and a steadfast commitment to the truth in all its forms. As patients in need of healing, we must be encouraged to uphold and live by truth and to practice personal integrity, honesty, and adherence to the teachings we consider holy scripture in order to combat the many deceptions of "the one who leads the whole inhabited Earth astray."[24]

Thief

Jesus described Satan as a thief whose "purpose is to steal and kill and destroy."[25] The precursor to stealing is *covetousness*—earnestly desiring something that is not rightfully yours, often accompanied by a sense of entitlement. Lucifer coveted mankind's rightful domain of the earth and God's position as supreme ruler who is owed worship.

In the Christian faith, Satan is often depicted as the ultimate deceiver, a being whose identity is fluid and whose primary method of subversion involves the manipulation of names and identities. Because of this tactic, Satan is sometimes referred to as a "name thief," suggesting that he not only deceives others by changing his own name and appearance but also steals and corrupts the identities of others.

Names in biblical times held significant power and meaning, and to steal or change a name was believed to alter one's identity and destiny. This idea is exemplified in the story of Jacob, whose name was changed to Israel after wrestling with God.[26] The Bible provides numerous examples of Satan changing his own name and appearance to deceive others. The first instance occurred in the Garden of Eden, where Satan takes the form of a *nachash* (shining one) in order to deceive Eve.[27] The New Testament reinforces this image, for example, when the Apostle Paul asserts, "Satan disguises himself as an angel of light."[28]

The theme of Satan as a name thief also appears in various literary and cultural works, highlighting the enduring fascination with this aspect of his character. In John Milton's *Paradise Lost*, Satan is depicted as a master of disguise and deception, assuming various forms to achieve his goals. In more contemporary literature, the concept is explored in works such as C. S. Lewis's *The Screwtape Letters*. In this epistolary novel, a senior demon, Screwtape, advises his nephew, Wormwood, on how to corrupt a human soul whom he interestingly calls his "patient." The manipulation of identity and the distortion of reality are central themes, reflecting the idea that the Devil's power lies in his ability to deceive and confuse.

In contemporary discussions, the concept of Satan as a name thief can be seen in the context of identity theft in the digital age. The ease with which identities can be stolen and manipulated online echoes the traditional themes of deception and corruption. This modern parallel highlights the timeless nature of the fears and anxieties associated with losing one's identity to a malevolent force.

On a more fundamental level, Satan shows himself to be a thief, in that he has stolen mankind's God-given rights to freedom and dominion on the earth. By leading mankind into rebellion and sin, Satan has enslaved all of humanity, stealing our freedom.[29] He also stole the title deed that granted humans dominion over the earth, and even though Jesus legally purchased it back by means of his sacrifice on the cross, Satan has claimed squatter's rights and now refuses to relinquish his unlawful occupancy. Part of the good news is that his day of eviction and subsequent incarceration is rapidly approaching. Until then, the enemy continues to, at times, successfully steal health, joy, peace, energy, focus, pleasure, and sleep, even from followers of God, in an attempt to render them ineffective soldiers in the cosmic war between good and evil. Realizing that unseen malevolent forces may be contributing to our health problems will hopefully make us aware of our need for a spiritual remedy to complement biological, psychological, and social treatments.

Tempter

The rise of technology and social media has introduced new dimensions to the concept of temptation. The constant bombardment of entertainment, information, advertisements, and opportunities for instant gratification are modern forms of temptation, echoing the traditional role of Satan as "the tempter" in the three Abrahamic faiths of Judaism, Christianity, and Islam. This concept of tempter reflects the belief that Satan's primary role is to entice humans into sin and away from God.

In the Old Testament, the earliest reference to Satan as tempter is found in the book of Genesis, where the serpent, traditionally interpreted as Satan, tempts Eve to eat the forbidden fruit by appealing to her curiosity and desire for knowledge.[30] The New Testament provides more explicit depictions.

First, in the account of Jesus's temptation in the wilderness, Satan attempts to derail Jesus's mission through a series of temptations, embodying the role of a cunning and persistent opponent.[31] Jesus's method of resistance to these is proposed as a model for people today to follow in their fight against illness.

A second significant reference is found in a letter from the Apostle Paul, in which he expresses concern that "the tempter" might have enticed the church members in Thessalonica, potentially undermining their faith and leading them astray.[32]

At this point, it is necessary to differentiate between the term *trials* and the term *temptations*. Scripture uses the Greek word *peirasmos* for trials, describing adversity sent or allowed by God to test one's character, faith, and holiness and thereby prove or disprove their devotion. Peirasmos has the connotation of something that disrupts the peace, comfort, and happiness in one's life. These tests are common to all mankind, and although difficult to varying degrees, they are never more than one can bear.[33] Trials rightly faced are actually beneficial to the person tested, but when wrongly met, they become temptations to evil. When we respond to adversity by turning to God in faith, we can successfully endure a trial, growing stronger in the process.[34] Conversely, if we respond with disobedience or doubt God, the trial becomes a temptation, which can lead to sin, giving spiritual enemies legal rights to oppress us further.

Essentially, Satan wants to turn God's tests that lead to righteousness into temptations that lead to evil. The "first Adam" that God created in his image and placed in his garden failed his test of righteousness, but "the second Adam," God's Messiah who came from heaven, passed his test in the wilderness, proving his righteousness.[35] God tests, but he does not tempt humans. It is Satan who tempts humans to be drawn away from the narrow spiritual path by means of their lust for possessions, power, prestige, accolades, accomplishments, relationships, and experiences.[36]

Tests always involve external circumstances, such as sickness or disease. Ruachiatry proposes that patients look at these difficult tests as opportunities for growth emanating from their higher power's permissive will, knowing that they can grow their faith, perseverance, and endurance amid their suffering. As patients grow stronger, they can face greater foes and become increasingly useful as a tool God can use to accomplish his larger kingdom objectives. Suffering in this fallen world is an inevitable fact, even for adopted children of God, so patients must place it in its proper perspective, knowing their current suffering "is nothing compared to the glory he will reveal to us later," according to Scripture.[37]

The key is for patients not to internalize their test but instead to give it to God, who promises strength, endurance, and a peace that surpasses human understanding and rises above adverse circumstances.[38] If, on the other hand, patients internalize the test of adversity they face, it becomes a temptation, kindling a small fire of lust ready to explode when the fiery darts of the adversary inevitably get shot in.[39]

Although no one likes trials, they are common to the human experience, so it is necessary for patients to understand their purposes. Christian pastor John MacArthur has suggested that there are eight purposes behind the trials God sends or allows. The first purpose is to reveal the strength of our faith or the lack thereof.[40] The second purpose is to humble us, as seen in the example of the Apostle Paul's thorn in the flesh.[41] The third purpose is to wean us from worldly possessions and interests.[42] The fourth purpose is to call us to an eternal hope, making us long for our glorification and for heaven, where our true treasure resides.[43] The fifth purpose is to reveal what we really love and value in life.[44] The sixth purpose is to teach us to value the blessing of God that comes from our obedience in the midst of the trial. Next, trials enable us to help others amid their own suffering, lending credence to the old adage that you cannot give someone something you do not yourself have.[45] Finally, God-ordained tests enable us to develop enduring strength for greater usefulness in the kingdom of God.[46]

In the words of nineteenth-century Scottish Baptist minister Alexander Maclaren, "Temptation says, 'Do this pleasant thing; do not be hindered by the fact that it is wrong.' Trial says, 'Do this right and noble thing; do not be hindered by the fact that it is painful.'"[47]

You and I choose which one we embrace.

Ruler of the World

The title "ruler of the world" conveys Satan's dominion over earthly realms and his influence over human affairs. As a beautiful, magnificently gifted, and anointed high-ranking angel, who before his rebellion was the pinnacle of God's created spiritual beings, Lucifer was accustomed to being in a position of leadership and was likely admired and revered by his fellow elohim. But, despite God's decree that those who desire to be great must humble themselves and serve others, when God created his physical human family, Lucifer's pride simply would not allow him to serve his younger, seemingly inferior, physical siblings. He regarded them as rivals to exterminate rather than family to love and help.[48]

Lucifer's personal ambition and self-will were set in opposition to the will of God. Before he tempted Adam and Eve with the promise of Godlike status through eating the forbidden fruit, Satan had already resolved to exalt himself, build his own kingdom, enshrine himself as its ruler, and become like the Most High.[49] The five "I will" statements of Satan recorded by the prophet Isaiah clearly show Satan exercising his self-will in rebellion to God's will. This stands in stark contrast to the Messiah's "Thy will be done" statements and his subsequent submission to God's will by voluntarily dying on a Roman cross.[50]

Mankind's Fall enabled Satan to have legal right to the title deed of the earth, formerly held by Adam. With authority to function as god of this world, Satan set out to blind mankind to spiritual truths and make them slaves to their bodily appetites and the world system he was building.[51] Over the millennia, up until today, some of these slaves would become willing servants of their "prince of the power of the air," because of his empty promises to grant them wealth, fame, and power in return for their service to the kingdom of darkness.[52] These once-exalted servants of his learn, in time, the hard lesson that Satan is the master of the bait and switch. The riches in Satan's kingdom are temporal, whereas the riches in God's kingdom are eternal. While a select few are exalted, the majority of his enslaved subjects toil in futility and have little impact during the shortened lifespan they endure on this earth.

Scripture informs us that Satan persuaded perhaps up to one-third of the heavenly angels to follow him in rebellion. Furthermore, in later Jewish literature, the idea emerged that three angelic rebellions described in the Old Testament were interconnected under Satan's command. Satan came to be viewed as the leader of a large demonic force made up of three groups: fallen angels, the disembodied spirits of the Nephilim giants, and minor deities assigned to the seventy nations scattered after the Tower of Babel incident.[53] Hence, it is clear that Satan has a worldwide kingdom with numerous powerful fallen angels in his demonic army.

In the New Testament, when facing temptation in the Judean wilderness, Jesus did not correct Satan when he told Jesus that the kingdoms of the earth were his to give to anyone he pleased.[54] This is because, surprisingly, Satan was telling the truth for once. In the Gospel of John, Jesus referred to Satan as the "ruler of this world" three times.[55] However, Jesus went on to declare that it was time for him to judge this world and drive out its ruler. The ruler of the kingdom of darkness was ultimately defeated and stripped of his authority through Jesus's mission, but in keeping with his prideful character, he refused to vacate his throne. In time, Satan will be forcefully removed by the rightful King when he returns.

Early church fathers, such as St. Augustine of Hippo, grappled with the implications of Satan's dominion over the world. While Augustine acknowledged Satan's influence and power, he argued that it is allowed by sovereign God's permissive will and ultimately serves God's greater plan of salvation. The Protestant Reformation brought new interpretations, with Martin Luther famously describing the world as a battleground between God and Satan. This reflected his belief in the pervasive nature of sin and the Devil's influence in both individual peoples' lives and in world affairs.

The notion of Satan as the ruler of the world can also be applied to contemporary issues, such as the corrupting influence of governmental power and systemic evil. Knowing there is a powerful, intelligent, evil force running the world from behind the scenes helps us understand how greed, injustice, and moral decay can pervade societies. This knowledge also helps solidify peoples' belief that there is a metaphysical dimension to human corruption with the hidden hand of malevolent spiritual forces providing undue influence. For example, it is plausible that Satan is the author of governmental systems that subvert individual freedom and promote authoritarianism, as seen in both fascism and communism. The founder of communism, Karl Marx himself, seems to confess this fact in his poem "The Fiddler":

Till heart's bewitched, till senses reel:
with Satan I have struck my deal.
He chalks the signs, beats time for me,
I play the death march fast and free.[56]

The sooner patients come to realize that they are foreigners living in an occupied territory ruled by a ruthless tyrant, unwittingly embroiled in an invisible spiritual war between good and evil, the better off they will be in their fight against their physical and mental maladies.

Destroyer

One of the more evocative and ominous titles attributed to Satan is "the Destroyer," a title that underscores his function as an evil force capable of ruin, the complete vanquishing of his foes, and even death.

This chapter has already demonstrated that Satan is a thief who comes to steal and a murderer who comes to kill, but what is meant by his intent to destroy? Satan hates his human rivals created in God's image to such a great degree that he wants to put an end to their very existence by keeping them from God, thereby ensuring that they join him in his final destination, the lake of fire.

If Satan fails to keep people from God, he then sets about to ruin them physically, emotionally, or spiritually, often employing sickness and disease as his means. The Apostle Peter describes Satan as a roaring lion who prowls around looking for someone to devour.[57] Lions most commonly stalk their prey before suddenly attacking, which causes the prey to panic and disperse. This dispersion allows the lions to isolate and attack weaker or slower individuals, just as physical or mental illness tends to socially isolate patients. And when lions are done with their prey, the devouring is so complete that only the skeletal remains are left.

In the book of Revelation, Satan is given the name *Abaddon* in Hebrew, and *Apollyon* in Greek, both of which mean "destroyer."[58] This reference explicitly links Satan with the act of total destruction, portraying him as the leader of demonic hordes allowed by

God's permissive will to wreak havoc upon the earth during the end times, prior to the Messiah's triumphant return. These demonic forces released from the bottomless pit are likened to locusts, insects that are known to totally destroy all vegetation in their path. The Destroyer is described as their king who gives them marching orders. Revelation says that Satan will work at first behind the scenes on the world stage, influencing leaders of the nations, and then openly when he eventually possesses and controls the one world leader called the Antichrist.

Early Christian theologians, such as Irenaeus and Origen, emphasized Satan's role in bringing about spiritual and physical ruin, which they believed to be a reflection of his opposition to God's creative and life-giving power. The medieval theologian Thomas Aquinas further elaborated on Satan's role as the Destroyer with his view that Satan's destructive acts were a deliberate attempt to corrupt God's creation and thus undermine the divine order.[59]

In the contemporary world, there are many other ways the Devil can cause destruction. For example, he can destroy people financially by enticing them to go into debt to purchase things that will not provide lasting joy. He can destroy families by means of alcohol and drug abuse, infidelity, anger and bitterness, and by fostering confusion about each member's role. Satan especially hates the family, because it was the foundation of civilization ordained by God from the very beginning. According to Scripture, because God created the family, he alone has the right to define its parameters as a covenant between one man and one woman until death. Satan has tried to destroy this foundation by his attempts to redefine the family.

Additionally, the Devil has tried to destroy the future of humanity in general in several ways. One I see often in clinical practice is the sowing of gender confusion among today's youth, leading some of them to receive medical treatments and surgeries that permanently alter their ability to conceive in the future. Other means include ending the lives of babies in the womb by abortion and cutting short the lives of young men and women via warfare. Thus, in the context of global issues, such as political unrest, war, environmental destruction, transgenderism, abortion, and societal decay, the archetype of Satan as the Destroyer remains relevant as a symbol of humanity's capacity for self-destruction under the sinister influence of its powerful spiritual adversary.

Serpent and Dragon

As discussed in Chapter 4, the biblical book of Genesis describes the first created woman conversing with a spiritual being called *nachash*, a Hebrew word that can be translated as "shining one," but which is most often translated in English Bibles as "serpent." Clearly Eve was not speaking with a literal serpent, as snakes lack the mental capacity and physical attributes—the type of palate, tongue, lips, vocal cords, and lung capacity—to both understand and generate speech. Because a literal interpretation is obviously scientifically ludicrous, many modern, educated people dismiss the creation account of Genesis altogether or see it as allegorical, similar to the Hindu creation myth in which the world held up on the back of a giant turtle.

But before we condemn the story of Genesis as ludicrous and likewise condemn Eve as being foolish enough to converse with an obviously evil serpentine being, a closer examination of the text informs us that, as Dr. Michael Heiser pointed out, the *shining one* definition of *nachash* likely conveys that the being was of a divine nature and that he could dispense divine information to Eve.[60] The biblical account does not state that Eve was surprised or alarmed by this being. Instead, she seems somewhat at ease, as if she had perhaps been accustomed to interacting with spiritual beings other than God or had even interacted with the nachash before. Eve was in all likelihood fooled by the enemy's appearance of shining beauty and his superior knowledge. Dazzled by these, it was likely only a matter of time before she bought his cunning lies.

Hence, the serpent in Genesis is symbolic of Satan's cunning and subtlety. Venomous snakes often lie hidden prior to suddenly striking their victims, so it is easy to see why many ancient cultures viewed them as a symbol of evil. But ancient cultures often had a dual representation of serpents as symbolizing both evil and wisdom, and this seems to fit the case in the biblical narrative as well.

According to Chad Bird in his article "The Devil in the Details of the Old Testament: Is Satan in the Hebrew Bible?," the non-canonical writings of Jewish thinkers and scribes, during the span of roughly four centuries between the closing lines of the Old Testament and the birth of Jesus in Bethlehem, offer us a valuable insight into how the earliest interpreters understood the serpent of Genesis—a figure whose identity, in time, would be unmasked.[61]

In texts such as *Wisdom of Solomon*, we read that "through the devil's envy, death entered the world," a direct echo of Genesis Chapter 3.[62] Though the serpent is the actor in the garden, these writers recognized the true voice behind the hiss—the enemy of life itself. Likewise, *The Life of Adam and Eve* does not mince words: it is the Devil who deceived Eve, leading her "to eat of the unlawful and forbidden tree."[63] These intertestamental sources point toward a spiritual culprit, pulling back the veil on what the Old Testament narrative only hints at.

By the time we arrive at the New Testament, the mask is off. The book of Revelation speaks with piercing clarity: "The great dragon was hurled down—that ancient serpent called the Devil, or Satan, who leads the whole world astray."[64] Here, the serpent and the dragon are not competing images but complementary ones. As serpent, Satan infiltrates quietly, weaving lies into the hearts of God's people like poison into water—subtle, calculated, nearly invisible. As dragon, he emerges in his fullness—an open destroyer, wreaking havoc, breathing chaos, and opposing all that is holy.

This is the enemy we face: at once deceptive and destructive, a master of both whisper and war. The Apostles understood this. When they read Genesis, they did not see a mere reptile slithering through Eden's brush—they recognized the serpent as a manifestation of Satan. They saw the dark intelligence behind this architect of the Fall through the lens of spiritual warfare. Today, the serpent still speaks. The dragon still roars. But we are not left defenseless in this cosmic war. The Great Physician has entered the fray—not only to heal our wounds and empower us, but to eventually crush the head of the serpent once and for all.

The Reality of Spiritual Warfare and the Devil's Destiny

There are many other names used for mankind's greatest spiritual enemy, but space in this context does not permit an exhaustive exposé on the subject. I have included the names I felt most relevant to the subject matter of this book.

The primary point here is that the Devil is neither a joke nor an allegory—he is a real and very powerful opponent, who should not be underestimated. Satan's three most prominent character traits are narcissistic pride, deceitfulness, and rebelliousness. He's at war with God, whom he is unable to get to directly, so he targets God's beloved human children. We humans must realize that we are in a fight, decide to take a stand and resist, and then become well-trained in the weapons of spiritual warfare.

The Devil holds many seemingly unfair advantages against us in this cosmic war. He is in charge of the world and its systems. He has a vast army with a battle plan, possesses supernatural powers, has numerous plausible lies and a massive propaganda machine to broadcast them, and has a worldwide surveillance system comprised of other malevolent spiritual beings. He is an older, wiser, more powerful enemy who is either disguised or invisible and who injures us, often before we even know we are in a fight.

It seems like the fight is fixed and that the odds are stacked against us. However, if we, as patients, identify our higher power, submit our lives and our will to him, heal from the past wounds we have incurred in the spiritual war, and diligently seek the omnipotent God, we will find victory, because the new Spirit of God now living in us is far greater than the spirit who lives in the world.[65] Satan is a defeated-but-dangerous foe who will, like a cornered predator, become increasingly unhinged as the day of his expulsion and incarceration approaches.

We need to understand Satan's ultimate fate.

It is a common misconception in our modern culture that Satan will reign as king in hell, presiding over the never-ending party filled with beautiful people, sex, drugs, and rock and roll. The biblical truth is that hell is an "everlasting fire prepared for Satan and his angels" as eternal punishment for their rebellion.[66] It is not a party by any stretch of the imagination. In seven places, the Bible uses the phrase "weeping and gnashing of teeth" to describe what will occur there.[67] Modern people have difficulty believing that a good God would send any human being to hell, but the truth is that no one is good, no one seeks after God, and all have sinned and fallen short of his perfect standard.[68] Additionally, what many neglect to consider is that not only is God good, but he is also just. It would be against his very nature to allow crimes to go unpunished. And since, as Scripture says, "the wages of sin is death,"[69] and all humans are born with a sin nature bent away from God,[70] we as a species are in big trouble. But God does not desire anyone to perish in the fire that he originally made for the fallen angels.[71]

Although Lucifer planned to ascend to the highest position of authority, God cast him down to earth as "a profane thing."[72] Jesus himself recounted that he "saw Satan fall like lightning from heaven."[73] This great fall of the mighty angel is a harbinger of his final fate, which is Gehenna, the lake of fire, the ultimate hell, where, Scripture says, "the maggots never die and the fire never goes out."[74] Every human is given the opportunity to avoid this same fate through Jesus's payment on the cross for their sins.

8

DEMONS: AGENTS OF CHAOS

Our policy, for the moment, is to conceal ourselves. Of course, this has not always been so. We are really faced with a cruel dilemma. When human beings disbelieve in our existence, we lose all the pleasing results of direct terrorism, and we make no magicians. On the other hand, when they believe in us, we cannot make them materialists and skeptics—at least not yet.

—UNCLE SCREWTAPE IN C. S. LEWIS'S
THE SCREWTAPE LETTERS

Introduction: Unmasking the gods

In a protracted ground war, foot soldiers are a necessity, and the more the better. Here is where demons come into play in our invisible cosmic war. They are Satan's "angels," malevolent, rebellious spirit beings who follow their leader's commands like any devoted soldier.[1]

Before explaining their role in the conflict, we must first define what demons are and what they are not, because there are many common misconceptions propagated by both Christian tradition and Hollywood machinations. As my pastor used to say, "It's not wise to think there's a demon around every corner—it's probably more like every other corner."

C. S. Lewis once said that many humans make one of two possible errors regarding demons: "One is to disbelieve in their existence. The other is to believe, and to feel an excessive and unhealthy interest in them."[2] Therefore, the information on demons in this chapter consists of what I consider to be the bare essentials to knowing our invisible-but-very-real enemies. I also echo Lewis's warning to the reader against unhealthy preoccupation with these supernatural villains.

Let's start with the basics.

Demons are not ghosts.

In fact, in the Judeo-Christian worldview, there is no such thing as ghosts, despite a massive Hollywood film industry telling us otherwise. Don't get me wrong; I do believe that demons at times masquerade as deceased humans, but we must remember that they are at their core liars bent on deception.

Nearly all cultures in history have held belief in malevolent spiritual beings, which modern people often call *demons*—a term originating from the Greek *daimōn*, meaning "deity, a divine power that acts as an influence in the world." Non-Western cultures, such as those in Asia, Africa, and Indigenous tribes, hold beliefs in evil spirits. For example, in Hinduism, Asuras are power-seeking deities who are often in conflict with the more benevolent devas. The demon Ravana in the ancient Indian epic, Ramayana, is a notable example of an Asura. In Buddhism, too, there are demonic beings, such as Mara, who tempted the Buddha by presenting obstacles to enlightenment. Likewise, traditional African religions often describe trickster spirits and malevolent ancestor spirits who can cause harm if not properly appeased.

In antiquity, the term *demon* generally had a neutral connotation and could refer to good or bad spiritual entities, all of whom were considered highly intelligent by nature. Belief in these entities is as old as civilization itself, dating back at least to the Fertile

Crescent of Mesopotamia. Ancient Sumerian writings show the culture's belief in malevolent entities they called *utukku* and *edimmu*, who were believed to cause disease, misfortune, and chaos. Later, Assyrian, Babylonian, and Canaanite cultures expanded on these beliefs and developed their own complex mythologies to explain evil and the rituals to appease or even exorcise these entities. Furthermore, the ancient Egyptians believed in a myriad of spiritual beings who could influence the world in both positive and negative ways. Apophis, for example, was believed to be an evil serpentine being who opposed the gods of Egypt.

Beliefs about these early Near Eastern evil beings influenced the later Israelite culture's understanding of demons, which evolved in the period between the Old and New Testaments. While specific references to demons are relatively sparse in the Old Testament, the ancient Israelites certainly had a belief in and fear of malevolent spiritual beings. While the Hebrew Tanakh speaks much more about angels than it does about demons, it occasionally references evil spirits, such as the one that tormented King Saul, causing depression and anxiety.[3] In fact, the Old Testament only uses the term *demons* in three passages, when the people of the nation Israel are chastised for making sacrifices to these malevolent spiritual beings.[4]

Ancient Israelites believed that the omnipotent creator God was a Spirit who dwelled in the spiritual realm, which humans could no longer perceive with their physical senses. The prophet Isaiah, who was supernaturally transported to the very throne room of God, described this spiritual realm where God resided as incredibly vast, so much so that he contrasts it with the physical creation, describing the latter as a mere tent made of thin cloth spread out before God's throne.[5]

According to the Hebrew Old Testament, because God desired a family, he first created a myriad of spiritual beings to inhabit his vast spiritual realm with him.[6] Created spiritual beings, including eventual fallen ones, have personality—that is, they are unique individuals with intelligence, will, and emotions. God wanted all his created family members to obey and serve him out of love and gratitude rather than compulsion. Hence, the members of God's spiritual family apparently also have freedom to choose to follow their self-will or God's will, just like the created members of God's physical, human family. According to the book of Genesis, God did not create a host of evil spirit beings, just as he did not create a Devil. In fact, all that God created was "good," and so his angels were not only created good but also holy, as they are described many times in Scripture. The term *angel* is more a job description of spiritual created beings than a title. They were originally created to serve as ministering spirits and occasionally messengers who reflect and magnify God's glory.[7]

Some time later, the angels watched as God created a completely different and unique physical realm, the natural universe, including the planet Earth, followed by creation of a unique human family having both a physical and spiritual nature. Humans were created to live eternally on this earthly realm, to populate it and rule over it. Death only came into the world as a consequence of mankind's rebellion toward God. Once mankind sinned, the species was destined to die a physical death and return to the dust of the earth.

Mankind's spirit, on the other hand, would not endlessly roam the earth upon death but rather go to one of two places—the spiritual realm called heaven, or the spiritual underworld called Hades, a temporary abode of the dead. Hades ostensibly functions as jail, a holding pen where the guilty await their day in court to be sentenced by the righteous Judge when he returns for his second coming. At this time, he will sentence both the unrepentant humans and the rebellious angels to spend eternity in the hellish prison, Gehenna, otherwise referred to as the lake of fire. This hell of eternal fire and torment was created for the rebellious angels who sinned, not for human beings, but they will nevertheless end up there unless they accept God's terms of peace.

The Hebrew Bible tells how these created, ministering spirits became malevolent enemy spirits by describing three angelic rebellions—one by Satan in the Garden of Eden, a second by a group of angels who left their proper domain to somehow mate with human women, and a third by angels who encouraged mankind after the great flood to make a name for themselves, build a tower to heaven, and disobey God's command to fill the earth. A brief description of each follows.

Angelic Rebellion #1

God is by nature omnipresent and thus desired to live among his created physical family. The initial overlap between the two realms allowed a degree of interaction among their inhabitants and with God himself, a very different circumstance from what we experience today. God not only lived among his created physical family but also conversed with them regularly, face-to-face. This is described in Genesis, which says God walked and talked with Adam and Eve in the midst of the garden before the Fall.[8] Likewise, the first humans apparently could also interact with other spiritual beings, as recounted in Eve's conversation with the supernatural nachash, the metaphorical serpent.

The first rebellious exercise of self-will occurred in the Garden of Eden by God's prideful first adversary, the nachash, who in later biblical writings morphed into the very embodiment of evil known as Satan. When this luminous guardian cherub tempted mankind to doubt God's Word and disobey his decree to not eat from the tree of the knowledge of good and evil, a state of chaos and depravity infiltrated God's formerly good creation.

Angelic Rebellion #2

At some point later, others among the innumerable elohim also made a conscious, willful decision to rebel against the Creator God and instead follow Satan. Because they exercised their own self-will against God's will, some of these beings became rebellious fallen angels. Genesis Chapter 6 describes this second angelic rebellion as a group of "the sons of God" who left their proper domain to satisfy their lust for the human women they found so beautiful by taking them sexually. As a result, Scripture says, "In those days, and for some time after, giant Nephilites lived on the Earth, for whenever the sons of God had intercourse with women, they gave birth to children who became the heroes and famous warriors of ancient times."[9]

With this second rebellion against God, the fallen angels demonstrated that they clearly shared the agenda of their leader Satan—they wanted to participate in human affairs and be worshipped as gods rather than serve their fellow image-bearers of the Most High God. Because they had the advantages of native intelligence and accumulated knowledge and wisdom from their thousands of years of existence, these rebel angels likely viewed their human siblings as inferior and refused to serve them as God had ordained. Desiring to create their own family, they fathered offspring who would become the earthly rulers of Satan's world. Some scholars postulate that the rebels' other desire was likely to corrupt the genetics of mankind to such an extent that God's recently revealed plan to bring forth a redeemer born of a woman would become impossible.

Whereas the rebellion in Eden was the initial cause of depravity, this second rebellion was the cause of the proliferation of depravity as, according to Second Temple Jewish apocryphal literature, these powerful fallen angels dispensed forbidden divine knowledge to mankind, ostensibly to curry humans' devotion, but ultimately to bring about their doom.

Some scholars have suggested that these unnatural offspring were the demigods and Titans spoken of in Greek mythology, such as Hercules, Achilles, and Perseus. We know from the entire counsel of God in the Bible, and from the testimony of the destruction of Sodom and Gomorrah in particular, that God views sexual sin as especially abominable. Both the Apostle Peter and Jude, the half brother of Jesus, stated that God therefore harshly judged these "angels who sinned" by sentencing them to a place called *Tartarus* in Greek, essentially a deep, impenetrable jail beneath Hades, often alternatively referred to as "the abyss."[10]

The apocalyptic Jewish literature of the intertestamental period served as a catalyst in the evolution of Hebrew demonology in several ways. First, apocalyptic texts such as the *First Book of Enoch* elaborated on the origin and nature of demons, suggesting they were evil, disembodied spirits of the deceased giant Nephilim, a Hebrew term meaning "fallen ones." These Nephilim were the offspring of the sons of God and human women described in Genesis Chapter 6. According to this non-scriptural book, after the abominable Nephilim hybrids were destroyed in the great flood, their spirits became malevolent entities condemned to roam the earth seeking embodiment and desiring to harm humanity. Their spirits could not return to God upon death since they were not originally created by God. The *First Book of Enoch* describes it this way:

And now, the giants, who are produced from the spirits and flesh, shall be called evil spirits upon the earth, and on the earth shall be their dwelling. Evil spirits have proceeded from their bodies; because they are born from men, [and] from the holy Watchers is their beginning and primal origin; [they shall be evil spirits on earth, and] evil spirits shall they be called. As for the spirits of heaven, in heaven shall be their dwelling, but as for the spirits of the earth which were born upon the earth, on the earth shall be their dwelling. And the spirits of the giants afflict, oppress, destroy, attack, do battle, and work destruction on the earth, and cause trouble: they take no food, [but nevertheless hunger] and thirst, and cause offenses. And these spirits shall rise up against the children of men and against the women, because they have proceeded [from them].[11]

Additionally, this intertestamental Jewish literature conceptually unified the three angelic rebellions described in the Old Testament by first recognizing Satan as head of a vast demonic army comprised of the fallen angels, the demonic disembodied spirits of the deceased Nephilim giants, and the lesser "gods" allotted to the seventy dispersed nations in the judgment following their attempt to build the tower at Babel.[12] The New Testament understanding of demons was significantly influenced by this non-inspired, extra-biblical Second Temple Jewish literature, such as the *First Book of Enoch*, which provides a much more detailed depiction of demons than that of the Old Testament.

The New Testament depicts Jesus frequently encountering and exorcising demons, and the text uses the same Greek term, *daimonion*, to refer to these evil, unclean spirits that is used in the Greek translation of the Old Testament, the Septuagint. By the time of the writing of the New Testament, the understanding of demons had evolved to recognition of them as agents of chaos in opposition to God's created order. Hence, demons in the New Testament are often depicted as causing physical and mental afflictions, promoting idolatry, and leading people astray from God's commandments. In the Gospels, Jesus's authority over demons demonstrates his purpose to restore the divine order by defeating the agents of chaos and destroying the works of the Devil.[13]

Angelic Rebellion #3

The famous story of the Tower of Babel, described in Chapter 4, is the precursor to the third divine rebellion. After the Creator judged the world with the great flood, sparing only Noah and his family, God reiterated the Edenic commandment to multiply and spread out over the earth. But as the people spread east, they settled instead in the plain of Shinar, where Noah's great-grandson, Nimrod, a satanically influenced rebel against God, founded Babylon. Nimrod's attempt to unite the population and build a tower in an effort to ascend into the divine domain prompted God to scatter the people, confuse their language, and assign spiritual members of the heavenly host to govern the resulting seventy nations on his behalf.[14]

The book of Daniel describes these angelic overseers of the various nations as "governors" or "princes." These divine beings, who were tasked with carrying out just governance of the nations that were allotted to them, eventually rebelled and began extending patronage to the people in exchange for their worship. For their refusal to obey God's decree that they govern justly on his behalf, God condemned these rebellious supernatural princes to death.[15] God made a covenant with one man of great faith, Abraham, whose descendants would become the great nation of Israel, chosen by God to be his separate and holy portion of the world. God, in turn, expected his people to worship him alone as the sovereign leader of their theocracy and to be a light to the scattered nations, drawing humanity back to God.[16] In essence, God allotted the seventy nations to other lesser "gods" while keeping Israel for himself.

Once the Israelites were freed from more than 400 years of captivity in Egypt, they found themselves surrounded by nations governed by these rebellious spiritual beings, or "gods," who were hostile to Yahweh and his chosen people. Although God had forbidden the Israelites to worship any other gods, including those who ruled over other nations, during the Israelites' wilderness journey following their exodus from Egypt, they defied God by worshipping some of the other nations' spiritual overseers, who were actually territorial demons. These governing, lesser gods, whom Moses referred to in Hebrew as *Shedim* (false gods), sowed chaos by inciting wars against Israel and seducing the Israelites to worship them instead of the Most High.

This third angelic rebellion, more than 3,500 years ago, threw God's created order into chaos, enabling Satan to extend his influence over the nations of the world in opposition to God's plan. The resulting spiritual warfare between the holy angels and the numerous spirit beings who were given dominion over the nations of this world continues to this day. It also seems to be escalating.

Ever since this third rebellion, our demonic foes have influenced worldly, carnal humans to attempt to unite the entire world under one government without borders, devoted to one counterfeit religion, and led by one satanically possessed dictator in order to fight the final apocalyptic battle, Armageddon. One day, they will succeed.

The Hierarchy and Tactics of Demonic Foes

We know from the Bible that angels have some sort of hierarchy, likely based on their job description and their abilities. For example, the Bible describes the pecking order as cherubim at the top, followed by seraphim, archangels, and then ministering spirits. Demons, as fallen angels and counterfeiters of God, also have a hierarchy. According to the Apostle Paul, a few categories of evil spirits include *thrones, dominions, principalities*, and *powers*.[17] Just as there are many ranks within any military based on ability, skill, intelligence, and devotion, I believe this to be true of demons as well.

While there is no consensus among scholars as to the meanings of the demonic ranks to which Paul refers, my opinion is that *thrones* have the connotation of kingship and therefore, likely refer to the god of this world, Satan himself. *Dominions* or lordships likely refer to Satan's top generals, who have great authority. *Principalities* likely refer to the territorial princes of the nations, such as the Prince of Persia and the Prince of Greece referred to in the book of Daniel. Finally, *powers* may refer to the remaining sinister foot soldiers on the front lines, warring with humans. Lest we erroneously underestimate our demonic foes as tricksters or merely spooky ghosts, it is vital to recognize that even the lowest-ranking demons are referred to as *powers*.

While these malevolent spiritual beings are indeed a reality, they rarely manifest openly, and almost never as ostentatiously and flamboyantly as depicted on Hollywood's silver screen. Most people will never recognize an encounter with a demon, because our evil enemies prefer to work behind the scenes, employing guerrilla warfare. It wasn't always this way. The fallen angels given control of the seventy scattered nations wanted worship and, in ancient times, would openly display their power and grant riches, positions of power, and forbidden knowledge to their devotees. For example, adherents of ancient Mesopotamian religion believed that knowledge of a particular craft or skill was due to patron deities of the respective skill.[18]

After Jesus sent out his Twelve Apostles to heal and cast out demons, he then deliberately sent out seventy other followers, likely as a sign to the principalities over the seventy nations, which scattered after Babel, that the kingdom of God had indeed arrived. The demons must have been relieved that their initial fear—that Jesus's arrival would bring their immediate sentencing to the abyss—wasn't realized during his three-year earthly ministry. However, they must have been shocked later to realize that the crucifixion they helped orchestrate did not ultimately result in the death of Jesus but rather the death of mankind's sin. At the cross, Jesus disarmed these evil spirits and made a public spectacle of them.[19]

Crestfallen, humiliated, disarmed, and defeated, the strategy of the unclean spirits had to change after the crucifixion. So, after they retreated, licked their wounds, and regrouped, they reemerged as stealth guerrilla warriors. Knowing the countdown to their ultimate demise had begun, they realized that they could best retain some degree of power by running an undercover operation. Otherwise, people might recognize the testimony of believers and the Bible to be true, increasing the likelihood of their repentance, freedom from the kingdom of darkness, and unification against their demonic foes.

But despite demons' plans to work in a more clandestine fashion in modern times, people in certain vocations, such as law enforcement, missionary service, the clergy, and the medical and mental health professions, will sometimes experience manifestations due to the nature of their work. I have witnessed what I believe to be demonic manifestations on a handful of clinical occasions and many times heard testimonies from others about them. I believe I encountered a malevolent supernatural entity years ago, while my family and I were vacationing in Nicaragua and on several mission trips to Third World countries where open demonic manifestations are not uncommon. I firmly believe that when light illuminates very dark places, these demonic entities can and sometimes will manifest in order to intimidate, harass one to leave, or even overtly attack.

Some good news for those on God's side is that in this spiritual war, there are several rules of engagement our enemies are compelled to follow. First, demons cannot directly kill humans or interfere with human free will. Furthermore, demons may not harm anyone sealed by God's Spirit without permission from God or legal right through open doors of willful rebellion or gross negligence. I like to think of demons as spiritual parasites that are attracted to and feed on human emotions, especially fear, anger, and lust. In medical school, I learned that the body's amazing defense system successfully thwarts the majority of pathogenic parasites. But when a patient has a compromised immune system due to diseases such as AIDS or certain medications, parasites that the body normally fends off become what are called "opportunistic infections." Like parasites, demons are opportunists who need a host, so they invade the minds of humans who let down their defenses. This negligence essentially gives them the legal right to attack unwitting human victims. Patients must bring their intrinsic nature into concert with God's nature in order to drive out the infestation.

The Three Ways Evil Spirits Affect Humans

To round out this important chapter on the enemies of God and us, his created physical beings, let's briefly discuss the three primary ways evil spirits can affect humans: possession, oppression, and influence. The fact is that very few humans will ever actually encounter Satan himself for the simple reason that he is too important and busy running his kingdom of darkness. He is likely singularly concerned with influencing very powerful world leaders, and most of us simply do not qualify. I believe the same principle likely holds true for the dominions and principalities responsible for overseeing large territories and groups of people. The remaining powers and possibly the disembodied spirits of the Nephilim are likely the levels of demons that most people will encounter in their lives.

Demonic Possession

Although the spirits of the Nephilim offspring of fallen angels and human women are not specifically addressed in the Bible, they are believed by some to be lower-level thugs and bullies who often display bravado, arrogance, taunting, and utterances of blasphemous speech when they manifest, reminiscent of the giant Goliath slain by David. According to non-inspired extra-biblical texts from the Second Temple period (536 BC to 70 AD), these Nephilim spirits roam the earth seeking embodiment and may be the primary source of the occurrence of demonic possession, widely acknowledged by exorcists and demonologists alike to be an exceedingly rare but well-documented phenomenon.

Possession involves a spiritual entity taking complete control of one's body, and human victims of demonic possession display certain telltale characteristics, such as having hidden knowledge, a strong aversion to anything holy, the ability to speak foreign languages unknown to the individual, and extraordinary physical abilities. By definition, the one who creates is the owner and possessor of his creation unless it is sold, gifted to another, or stolen. Although created by God, mankind, because of sin, has been separated from God and turned over to pursue our own will, opening us up to demonic influence. God, in his grace, still loves his wayward human children and calls for us to turn from our rebellious ways back to him. Possession by unclean spirits can only occur in rebellious humans who have not accepted God's invitation to receive salvation and the restoration of their relationship with him. But even then, it is exceedingly rare, most commonly occurring in those who have completely sold out to the kingdom of darkness in a foolish deal to achieve temporary wealth, power, position, and fame, or in those who were either repeatedly willfully rebellious or spiritually neglectful as to allow the enemies legal rights to enter via "open doors" that will be addressed more thoroughly in Chapter 11.

While the idea of demonic possession has pervaded our culture, largely by means of Hollywood horror films such as *The Exorcist*, many people are surprised to learn that dramatic episodes of demonic possession are also described in the Bible. But there are no examples in Scripture of believers being possessed by a demon.

Furthermore, most theologians postulate that believers cannot be possessed, because the Spirit of God residing within them would not share residence with an unclean spirit.[20]

According to the biblical accounts, demonic possession can present with a wide variety of possible physical, emotional, behavioral, and spiritual symptoms. For example, some passages show that possession can cause physical ailments such as inability to speak, epileptic symptoms, and blindness when these physical impairments cannot be attributed to an underlying physiological problem.[21] Likewise, personality changes, depression, physical aggression, superhuman strength, immodesty, antisocial behavior, self-cutting, and perhaps the ability to share information that one has no natural way of knowing are possible emotional and behavioral manifestations of possession seen in the Bible.[22] In addition to these physical or emotional distinctions, certain spiritual attributes suggest the possibility of demonic influence, including a refusal to forgive and the belief in and spread of false doctrine.[23]

The most extensive biblical account involves an insane, violent homeless man possessed by demons, who lived naked among the tombs in the land of the Gadarenes.[24] When Jesus arrived in that area, the demons immediately recognized Jesus and acknowledged his authority over them. There was no battle or skirmish, as the mighty legion of demons that possessed this poor man cowered in fear; Scripture says they were "begging Jesus not to send them into the bottomless pit."[25] As soon as Jesus cast the demons out into a nearby herd of pigs that plunged off a cliff and drowned in the Sea of Galilee below, the man was said to be seen "sitting at Jesus's feet, fully clothed and perfectly sane."[26] This showed that the man's mental illness and subsequent bizarre behavior, aggression, and self-cutting were caused by the demonic possession.

It is important to note that nearly all, if not all, of these characteristics may have other explanations, so it is vital not to label every patient who has scientifically inexplicable physical or psychological symptoms as "demon possessed." Although most cases of psychosis or other severe mental illness are not the result of demonic possession or influence, some clearly are. My belief is that spiritual causes or contributions to any illness should be considered only *after* the influence of toxic substances and all biological and psychological causes have been ruled out by medical professionals.

Even though the man possessed by a legion of demons was a Gentile with a terrible past, he was so radically transformed that he amazingly became the very first missionary Jesus sent out. Even though after his exorcism he begged to go with Jesus, the homeless man obeyed Jesus's command, Scripture says, to return to his town and proclaim "the great things Jesus had done for him."[27] He obviously spread the word not only to his town but also throughout the ten-city region called Decapolis, because when Jesus later returned to that area, the townspeople brought a deaf and mute man to Jesus, knowing that he had the ability to heal.[28]

Demonic Oppression

As opposed to the rare phenomenon of possession, demonic oppression of humans is a ubiquitous phenomenon that is experienced by all but recognized by only a few. Fewer still know how to effectively fight their oppressors. Possession takes hold from the inside out, whereas oppression works its way from the outside in. Believers are not immune to oppression, but they have both the Spirit of God living within them and spiritual armor to help them fight back.

Oppression can present as harassment, in which patients' spiritual enemies orchestrate circumstances or influence other people to frustrate, hinder, or even harm them. But oppression can also present as outside mental influence that is construed by its victims as intrusive, unwanted, and often disturbing in nature. These thoughts are perceived as foreign, and due to their unrelenting obsessive character, they can be difficult to differentiate from certain psychiatric disorders, such as severe obsessive-compulsive disorder (OCD), for example. In my experience, when these thoughts are felt by the patient to be demonic or contain disturbing immoral or blasphemous content, the possibility of demonic oppression should be entertained after other causes have been ruled out and if symptoms are not responsive to traditional medical and psychological treatments.

I have seen numerous cases of treatment-resistant OCD in my clinic over the years, some of which had a very peculiar presentation of intrusive thoughts. One case involved a college student I'll call Jane, who presented with intrusive thoughts of sexually molesting children that had progressed to the point where she avoided situations in which she might encounter a child. She was otherwise an intelligent, well-adjusted young lady from a stable, intact home who identified as heterosexual and had no history of trauma or attraction to minors. Jane had undergone a prolonged course of cognitive behavioral therapy (CBT) and medical treatment with several serotonin reuptake inhibitors, the tricyclic antidepressant clomipramine, an atypical antipsychotic, and a six-week course of transcranial magnetic stimulation with only minor benefit.

While her emotions were a bit more regulated after treatment, the intrusive thoughts and images persisted and significantly impaired her functioning. In the course of taking a spiritual history, Jane said that while she was raised by Christian parents, she now identified as Wicca and looked to the earth for spiritual power. After solidifying a rapport with her, I gradually asked her more probing questions about how she came to practice Wicca. "So many Christians are hypocrites," she explained, "so I was looking for something else, and some friends introduced me to

Wicca . . . We're not witches—we just believe in harnessing the energy and spirit of the earth."

Over time, Jane and I came to agree that there may indeed be a spiritual component to her illness. I suggested she ask her higher power for help, and she enthusiastically complied. Unfortunately, she found no help there.

I challenged her to consider other higher powers that could possibly help. "Don't get hung up on religion or other people who profess certain beliefs," I encouraged her. "Search out the matter for yourself with an open mind, and make sure you are appealing to the highest power who might be able to help you with your illness."

Jane did the hard work most people do not, and her condition gradually began to improve. She became increasingly functional and was able to return to college after taking a semester off in the wake of her illness.

During one session, she appeared to be a completely different person—smiling and visibly calmer.

"The thoughts are almost completely gone," she said after informing me of her plans to return to college. "And when they do crop up, I have control over them and can dismiss them."

Almost as an afterthought, she then said, "Oh, by the way, I'm Christian again" and went on to explain how her search had led her back to her original beliefs and how she was excited to have a growing relationship with God through prayer, Bible reading, and a community of other Christians.

Demonic Influence

The final common way that demons affect people is by means of influence. Just as there are gradations in the degree of intoxication from a substance such as alcohol, there are also degrees of being under the influence of malevolent spirits. There can be complete transfer of ownership, as seen in rare instances of possession, as well as varying degrees of occupancy, depending on the nature, frequency, and duration of open doors. The battleground is the mind, so this influence can range from common whispered demonic suggestions and enticements to less common demonic obsessions and harassment to the complete mind control seen in possession.

People often open themselves up to demon involvement by the rebellious act of embracing some habitual sin or through idolatry (putting devotion to anything else above devotion to God), occultic involvement, drug or alcohol abuse that alters one's state of consciousness, feelings of bitterness, and transcendental meditation, to name a few examples. Our demonic foes have been observing humans for centuries and know well where our weaknesses lie. When unsuccessful at keeping people away from God, demons then attempt to nullify peoples' effectiveness on the battlefield by enticing them to get very entangled in the cares of the world system or to rebel against God by seeking to gratify their God-given desires in a context other than what God intended.

Discernment amid Spiritual Battles

The question remains: How can people differentiate between the invisible, clandestine work of the demonic and other difficult circumstances in life caused by happenstance, other people, or sickness?

First, there is no such thing as chance, because God is sovereign, and everything occurs as a result of him either decreeing it or allowing it. In all kingdoms, including the spiritual realm, there are rules of order and laws. Humans have been granted the freedom either to abide by the laws decreed by the King or to exercise their self-will. Satan acts as a ruthless prosecuting attorney, the accuser of the brethren, who has innumerable demonic policemen patrolling the earth. Just as it is foreseeable that something bad might happen if people do unwise things in the physical realm, such as play golf in a lightning storm or attempt to climb Mount Everest when they're old and out of shape, there are likewise natural consequences that hold true for those who act in defiance of God's laws. Simply put, sinning opens humans up to demonic influence, and habitual sin gives our spiritual enemies a foothold, which they gradually build into a stronghold in our minds.

Second, there is the question of whether other people treating us unjustly, rudely, or harshly may be a demonic attack. The majority of the time, humans are quite capable of reacting to others in a selfish and harsh manner without any need of help from demons. Because of this and the fact that these demonic encounters are not dramatic in nature, they are difficult to discern. But when people go by the letter of the law, so to speak, and their reaction or "punishment" tends to be far out of proportion to the "crime," extending no mercy to the alleged perpetrator, then there may be a spiritual influence behind the behavior.

For example, I recently woke early on a Saturday to drive up to the local Golden Pantry to treat myself and my family to their incredible breakfast biscuits. I pulled into a parking space and apparently parked on the line to my right because the car parked on my left had parked on the line between our spaces.

As I exited my car, a burly man pumping gas behind me yelled, "Hey! Who the hell do you think you are? Move your car [expletive]—nobody has room to park next to you!"

I was startled, but rather than arguing, I got back in my car and reparked six inches to the left. When I got out, he continued berating me and followed me halfway into the store.

Once inside, I stopped and prayed for protection and asked God to quench this man's anger, whatever its source.

He suddenly stopped, turned, and walked back to his truck. I responded in this fashion because years ago, I decided that there were only a few things in life worth fighting for, and my parking skills were not one of them. Could this man have just been having a bad day and chosen someone on whom he could take out his anger? That's certainly possible, but because of him reacting as merciless judge, jury, and potential executioner to my minor infraction, I wonder whether there might have been some spiritual influence behind his behavior.

In Scripture, Satan and his demons often employ their sons of disobedience—humans bent toward their will—to persecute others. The difficult trick is to refuse to react naturally, by returning evil for evil, and instead to respond supernaturally, by returning good for evil behavior. Rather than attacking the person, we ought to appeal to God to help us deal with the power behind their actions. Jesus demonstrated this when he famously addressed the Apostle Peter with "Get thee behind me, Satan," when Satan influenced Peter to entice Jesus not to follow through with his God-given mission.[29] Peter was not possessed—he was an Apostle, who became a pillar of the early Church. But Peter was influenced by Satan when he reacted emotionally to Jesus's statement, and Jesus successfully rebuked the spirit hiding behind his behavior and words rather than Peter himself.

Finally, regarding sickness, we should consider potential spiritual involvement when symptoms are unusual, chronic, and/or severe, despite appropriate lifestyle modifications and evidence-based, standard medical or psychiatric treatment. The Devil and his minions are powerful counterfeiters, who can mimic symptoms of known medical disease to cause harm and confusion.

Authority over Darkness

Demons have authority and power over humans who are enslaved citizens of the kingdom of darkness. But the good news is that, although humans battle against invisible, powerful, and malevolent spiritual adversaries, the God of the Bible is sovereign, and evil spirits can do nothing to humans who have submitted to and placed their faith in God unless God allows it through his permissive will.[30] Incredibly, believers are given positional authority over these evil spirits by God himself. "Look," Jesus assured his followers, "I have given you authority over all the power of the enemy, and you can walk among snakes and scorpions and crush them. Nothing will injure you."[31]

While no weapon formed against believers will prosper, make no mistake—weapons will still be formed against you if you side with God.[32] According to the Bible, humans are locked in a wrestling match with spiritual principalities and powers, and the Greek term used to describe it, *pale*, implies a physical fight to the death.[33] Humans must therefore never underestimate our spiritual enemies and must likewise realize that a believer's power and authority come from God alone, not from our own strength or efforts.

A biblical example of the prideful misuse of this imputed authority over demons is seen in the account of the seven sons of Sceva. In the first-century Asia Minor city of Ephesus, God was performing mighty miracles through the Apostle Paul to validate his message, including casting out demons. A Jewish chief priest named Sceva had seven sons who attempted to replicate exorcisms performed through the power and authority of God by stating the mantra, "In the name of the Jesus whom Paul preaches, I command you to come out."[34] This formula of invoking the name of Jesus seemed to work until one day they encountered a powerful demon who did not recognize their authority. The Scripture says:

> *But one time when they tried it, the evil spirit replied, "Jesus I know, and Paul I know about, but who are you?" Then the man with the evil spirit leaped on them, overpowered them, and attacked them with such violence that they fled from the house, naked and battered.*[35]

Several lessons can be learned from this account. One, don't pick a fight with demons—the fight will find you. Two, only believers with pure lives and strong faith wield the authority and power to successfully engage with these entities when the battle finds them. Three, believers must put on the full armor God graciously provides to protect them in the invisible spiritual war; rely on the power and authority of Jesus, who demonstrated power over demons; and regularly engage in practices of spiritual disciplines such as prayer, scripture reading, and corporate worship to resist demonic influence.

Awakening to the Covert Demonic Influences

Despite modern advances in science and technology, belief in demons persists across many cultures. As evil and depravity flourish in our world, many people today are awakening to the reality that we humans do not wrestle with flesh and blood but rather against very powerful spiritual enemies who seem to be increasingly more willing to step out from behind the veil. While time has marched on, and over the millennia, history has seen many evil empires rise and fall, one thing has remained constant—the demonic spirits behind them all.

Scripture offers evidence of this in Jesus's words about a malevolent spirit at work within the church in the ancient city of Thyatira, in present-day Turkey. He identified that spirit as the spirit of the evil, domineering queen Jezebel of Israel, who had died nearly 900 years prior. Addressing the church, Jesus said, "But I have this against you, that you tolerate the woman Jezebel."[36] Therefore, we must first identify the spirit behind the negative people and circumstances in our lives and then not tolerate it. This is difficult, since *tolerance* has recently become a buzzword that implies freedom and open-mindedness, when tolerance is, in fact, the sinister means by which evil spirits are voluntarily given control.

Once in control, those who fought so hard for tolerance surprisingly tend to become quite intolerant themselves. As the culture grows more secular and morally progressive, there is a growing tension between the moral absolutes and exclusive truth claims of Bible-believing Christians and the modern emphasis on relativism and inclusivity. Intolerance of Bible-believing Christianity today often manifests as social stigma, cultural marginalization, or pressure to conform to cultural norms. Many of those who proudly decorate their cars with the popular bumper sticker "Coexist," which displays religious symbols of seven different faiths, embrace relativistic or pluralistic worldviews and tend to reject Bible-believing Christianity's exclusive truth claims. We must realize that history clearly shows that societies that are overly tolerant of evil start to gradually label *good* as *evil* and *evil* as *good* before they inevitably crumble. Faithful followers of God, however, need not be afraid, for the outcome is not in doubt—God wins and will one day expose the forces that work behind the scenes to move the culture away from traditional moral values.

The questions that remain are:

Will you be on the winning side?

What role will you play in this cosmic battle: naive, civilian collateral damage or battle-ready soldier for good?

9

STRATEGIC INTEL PART I: THE BATTLE PLAN FOR THE NATURALLY BORN SLAVES

All warfare is based on deception.

—SUN TZU

Motive of Enslavement and Methods of Deception

I became a forensic psychiatrist in 2002, after completing a fellowship at the East Coast's federal maximum-security prison affiliated with Duke University and then passing the specialty board examination. During my fellowship, one of my main roles in performing court-ordered evaluations at the prison was to detect deception. In time, I became very good at it.

I specifically recall one court-ordered evaluation in which the inmate was accused of kidnapping someone and taking her across multiple state lines. The inmate in question made the legal defense that he was not responsible for his alleged crime because he claimed he had no recollection of his alleged violent kidnapping due to supposed dissociation, resulting from his assertion that he suffered from dissociative identity disorder, formally known as multiple personality disorder.

This inmate was a convincing actor, who I discovered just so happened to be very well-read on the subject of dissociative identity disorder, having checked out many books about the psychological malady from the prison library. But in observing him over four months, I noticed he would slip up at times and forget the role he was playing.

I learned during the course of my fellowship that time and thoroughness were two main keys to detecting deception. By the time my official report to the court was due, I was excited that I had an airtight case showing the inmate to be feigning mental illness, and I asserted that he was responsible for the crime of which he was accused and ready to return to court for further legal proceedings.

My physician supervisor during my forensic psychiatry fellowship, Dr. Bruce Berger, commented on my enthusiasm by jokingly saying, "Tom, you sure like to catch bad guys!" I sure do. My broadening knowledge of how to psychologically profile criminals along with my newfound spiritual beliefs were the likely reasons that thwarting history's ultimate bad guys' sinister plans has become one of my passions.

The Devil, as "the commander of the powers in the unseen world," knows full well that he and his demonic army cannot defeat the omnipotent creator God in their own power.[1] Therefore, although the Devil began an insurrection against God, his strategic battle plan now is against God's human children. His sinister battle plan is against *me and you*—body, soul, and spirit. We must realize that we are both the pawns and the prize in the invisible cosmic war.

Other faiths share this conceptualization of an evil, deceptive force battling against humans. For example, in Islam, Iblis (Satan) refused to bow to Adam and was cast out, vowing to lead humans astray. In Judaism, the *Yetzer Hara* (evil inclination) tempts humans to sin. Hinduism speaks of Maya, the illusion that veils the true nature of reality, and Buddhism warns of Mara, the tempter who tried to distract the Buddha from enlightenment.

In the Christian faith, although both highly intelligent and vastly knowledgeable, Satan is not all-knowing like God and therefore must always wait for God's progressive revelation in order to plan his next move in this war. Satan may have fired the first shot in the war, but God was not caught by surprise. Because of his omniscient foreknowledge, God had planned before the foundation of the world to send a human redeemer who would ultimately crush Satan and reverse the curse placed on all of physical creation due to mankind's rebellion. When God first revealed his plan in Genesis Chapter 3, Satan's initial countermove was an attempt to corrupt the seed of the woman with the seed of other rebellious angels so that this prophesied human redeemer could not be born in the first place.

God's successful military response, in turn, was to use a global flood to wipe out the resulting abominable hybrid offspring and the entire increasingly evil human race, except for eight people.[2] Although Satan was resoundingly defeated in this battle, he did not surrender. Satan always regroups, sowing chaos while waiting for another opportunity.

Because Satan is perhaps the most intelligent, powerful, and gifted of God's created beings in history and has vast human and demonic resources, the Apostle Paul warns that being ignorant of Satan's strategies gives him an additional advantage over us.[3] But, just as I learned to detect deception in inmates feigning mental illness in an attempt to evade responsibility for their crimes, you can also learn the schemes and plans the Devil employs in his fight against you.

How? By means of the truth revealed in holy scripture.

While time and thorough investigation are very important in detecting deception, the most crucial factor is having a tight grasp of the truth. Simply put, the more truth one knows, the easier it is to detect the lies of history's most notorious counterfeiter. US Secret Service agents will attest that the best way to recognize a counterfeit $100 bill, for example, is not by studying all the myriad ways criminals go about manufacturing fakes but by having an in-depth knowledge of what the real thing looks like. Satan longs to be like God, but the best the prince of darkness can offer to tempt people trapped in his world system is a flashy counterfeit religion that promises its adherents only passing pleasures and gratification of their natural appetites. The problem is that this type of gratification is unsatisfying, so no matter how many times people seek it out, they will never experience the permanent satisfaction that comes from God's truth, what he calls "the bread of life" and the "living water."[4] Because of their spiritual blindness, it is very difficult for these unsuspecting citizens of the kingdom of darkness to discern the difference between the counterfeit and the authentic.[5]

As demonstrated earlier, Satan is, at his core, a self-willed thief whose motive is murder and method is deception, a craft he has honed over thousands of years of observing human nature. The Devil, therefore, acts in accordance with his nature when he comes "to steal and kill and destroy," but I believe an additional goal of his as the ruler of a seized kingdom is to maintain the state of slavery into which his subjects were born. This state would enable Satan to control his subjects and ultimately destroy them by keeping them from God's rescue plan.[6]

The Devil's strategy has not changed over the centuries. With lies and deception, he hinders the dissemination of ultimate truth by attacking the words of God, the ways of God, and God's embassy in the world, the Church. His method of deception typically involves three strategies: concealment of his true feelings, intentions, and character; propaganda (promoting false ideas); and hiding the truth via sleight of hand, distraction, or camouflage.

When Satan tempted Adam and Eve to sin, mankind suffered spiritual death and enslavement to sin. Satan seized the title deed from its original owner and proceeded to build a kingdom of darkness to control his enslaved subjects. His kingdom still stands today and wields its power and influence throughout the world.

But there is another kingdom, God's Kingdom of Light, which is ruled over by a sovereign, all-powerful God who will have the final say. The citizens of his kingdom have been delivered from bondage by the acceptance of his truth, resulting in a supernatural spiritual rebirth.

Satan has a different strategic battle plan for the citizens of each of these two kingdoms. Exploring Satan's four overarching goals to enslave, steal, kill, and finally destroy humans in the context of mankind's spiritual journey will enable us to remain aware of his evil schemes and thus be better equipped to fight the spiritual war.

The Spiritual Journey

The metaphors of slavery, deliverance, wandering through the wilderness, and the eventual taking of the Promised Land resonate across various religious and philosophical traditions and provide a template of the four stages of life's spiritual journey. In Hinduism, the journey of the soul is seen as moving from the enslavement of ignorance (*avidya*) to knowledge (*vidya*), through the stages of life (*ashramas*), ultimately seeking the liberating deliverance of *moksha*. Buddhism describes the Noble Eightfold Path from suffering (*dukkha*) to enlightenment (*nirvana*), while Islam speaks of the straight path (*Sirat al-Mustaqim*) leading to paradise. The Exodus story of Judaism and Christian's journey to the Celestial City to find redemption in John Bunyan's novel *Pilgrim's Progress*, round out these archetypal motifs that encapsulate universal truths about the human condition and the pursuit of spiritual awakening. These stages offer insights into the challenges, transformations, and ultimate fulfillment encountered on the path to spiritual awakening. The Devil employs different strategies depending on where we are in our own spiritual journey.

The ultimate goal of the journey for each of us is to return to union with our transcendent higher power, what most faiths call *God*, and to reach our eternal destination, the Promised Land of a new heaven and a new earth without sin, sickness, suffering, or death. But the Devil has other ideas.

His primary goal is for us to remain stuck in the slave state into which we were born, which will result in the satisfaction of all of his objectives to enslave, steal, kill, and finally destroy God's created imagers.

Ideally, life's spiritual journey should move through the four stages that the ancient Israelites experienced: 1) slavery, 2) deliverance, 3) wandering, and 4) entrance into the Promised Land.

But sadly, the majority of people naturally born into the first stage of slavery remain there their entire lives, because the kingdom of darkness is set up to hide the light of truth that could enable their escape to freedom. It is also set up to indoctrinate and distract slaves, so they neglect or discount the importance of spiritual pursuits. Even if sojourners are fortunate enough to be freed, they still may get stuck in either of the next two stages in their spiritual journey as Satan both blinds them to truths he does not want them to know and entangles them in the world system he controls.

Phase 1 of the Spiritual Journey: Slavery

Slavery is an abominable, dehumanizing practice that is a blight on the history of the United States, in particular, especially because the country was established based on the principle of freedom. But the enslavement of Africans by other Africans, Europeans, and Americans was not new. Slavery has existed for thousands of years and historically was most often instituted when the peoples of tribes or nations conquered in war were captured by the victors. One of the many evils of slavery was that one could be born into it—if expectant parents were slaves, their baby would become a slave at birth.

Religious faiths have different perspectives on human nature. In Islam, humans are born pure (*fitrah*) but can be led astray by Shaytan. Judaism holds that humans have both good and evil inclinations (*Yetzer Tov* and *Yetzer Hara*) and must choose to follow God's law. Hinduism and Buddhism see humans as caught in the cycle of *samsara* due to *karma*, with the potential for liberation through spiritual practice. And according to the Christian interpretation of the Bible, all humans are unwittingly born slaves. But it was not this way in the beginning. Although God originally created mankind to be free, this freedom was relinquished when mankind rebelled from God in the Garden of Eden. Not only did everything become more difficult for humans because of the curse God put on the earth itself, but they also had to deal with a permanent and incurable infection of sin that the first of their race passed down to them.[7]

With God's creation, which was entirely good before it fell due to angelic and human rebellion, God intended to have two families, one human and one divine, working to bring about his will in two different but overlapping realms. He desired unity in diversity, one unified kingdom under the benevolent rule of one King, having created sons and daughters to help him administer his rule—not because he needed them but because he chose to share this responsibility with them.

When Satan stole the title deed to the earth from the first Adam, he founded a kingdom of darkness built upon subterfuge and lies to preserve the slave state into which all of its subsequent human citizens are born. To maintain this slave state, Satan employs five chief methods.

Method #1: Blinding the Minds of Unbelievers

Humans were created as beings composed of three parts—body, soul, and spirit—but original sin and the subsequent Fall led to the consequence of spiritual death.[8] From that time of history onward, all humans have been born with a body and a soul but a stillborn spirit.[9] Because their spirit is dead, they lack spiritual senses, making it relatively easy for the god of this world to control his slaves by keeping them blind to the spiritual truths that could set them free.

The Devil thus acts as the Wizard of Oz, hidden behind the curtain, programming humans' minds with his own false ideologies, materialism, and secularism, primarily by means of the propaganda arm of the world system he controls through media and entertainment. For example, the entertainment industry's progressive influence in moving our culture away from traditional morals and values can clearly be seen in the contrast between the moral outrage in 1958 when the hit song "Wake Up Little Susie" was released and the wide acceptance of the more recent hit song "W.A.P." The same can be said of the television and film industries, which have gradually desensitized the public to images of nudity, sex, and violence.

I would argue that this is all part of the strategy of mankind's powerful spiritual adversaries working directly behind the scenes or indirectly through their "children of disobedience." This strategy keeps the good news of the Kingdom of Light hidden, and only a few are curious enough to probe behind the curtain to find it.[10] Other faiths also suggest that spiritual enemies are working in a clandestine manner to keep mankind in darkness. In Islamic thought, Shaytan, a rebellious jinni akin to Satan, whispers evil suggestions (*waswas*) to humans, trying to lead them away from the truth. In Hinduism, Maya creates an illusion that makes the material world seem more real than the spiritual. Buddhism warns against the defilements (*kle-shas*) that cloud the mind and prevent enlightenment.

Method #2: Denying God

Dealing with this tactic of denying or distorting the divine is a shared challenge across religious faiths. For example, in Islam, Shaytan tries to make people forget God and become heedless, while in Judaism, the Yetzer Hara tempts people to idolatry or to doubt God's commandments. In Eastern religions, the concept of *avidya* (ignorance) leads to misunderstanding the nature of the divine or ultimate reality.

According to the Christian conceptualization, the Devil would ideally like his slaves to believe that God does not exist at all; however, this turns out to be quite difficult because Scripture states that only a few fools truly believe in their hearts that there is no God.[11] So, Satan's next best method is to prevent the seed of God's truth taking root in the hearts of humans and then to spread lies to them about God.

In his parable of the sower, Jesus explained that the sower is God, and the seed is his truth. The seed that lands along the path represents those who hear the message but do not understand it due to their spiritual blindness. Being by nature a thief, Satan comes and snatches it away, preventing the message from taking root in their hearts.

Since God does indeed exist, and Satan cannot kill him, the murderer tries to kill ideas about God and sow confusion about his true identity and character. One way the Devil goes about this is by attempting to kill God the Judge and magnify God the Lover. The enemy's attempts to kill the one rightful Judge appear very plainly in our culture today in the concept of "social justice" rising to pre-eminence above divine justice. Two of the favorite quotes today by enslaved children of the world are "judge not, lest ye be judged" and "God is love." But this tactic of taking a quote from Scripture completely out of context and using it to deceive is the same old trick the Devil employed in the Garden of Eden and also in the temptation of Jesus in the wilderness.

The truth is that God is *both* a righteous Judge and an unfailing Lover, not one or the other. While it is a Scriptural truth that God is love, God does not love everything and everybody. In fact, God hates sin and actually commands believers to not love certain things, such as the world system under Satan's control.[12] Unredeemed members of the human family desperately want there not to be a judge so that they can indulge their self-will in the world's pleasures without any responsibility or consequences. However, the same individuals hypocritically clamor for a righteous and good judge who does not allow crime to go unpunished when they or someone they care about is harmed.

Likewise, the Devil tries to kill the idea that God is holy and magnify the idea he is an indulgent Father who wants his human children to be happy above all else. The Devil's lie is, "You are all God's children, so a good and righteous Father would not send his kids to hell, because he is a God of forgiveness." First, not all humans are in fact his children. It is only to those who both believe and receive him that he grants "the right to become children of God" by adoption.[13]

While it is true that he created mankind in his image, that he loves us and does not want anyone to perish, God's high standard of holiness demands a certain caliber of conduct and thinking in his children. Far from being indulgent, Scripture teaches that God "disciplines those he loves, and he punishes each one he accepts as his child."[14]

Another one of the Devil's lies is "Since God gave you natural desires, such as those for food and sex, he wants you to satisfy them." Here again is Satan's subtle tactic of wrapping up something that is true within the package of a bigger lie. God does want mankind to have those desires fulfilled but only in their proper context, timing, and proportion. For example, sex is a wonderful gift to be enjoyed but only in the context between a man and a woman having entered the covenant of marriage. This belief is not widely held today, but God does not change as our societal norms do. Since God created sex, he alone has the right to define its boundaries and parameters. Holy Scripture teaches that the only way to be assured that God will grant humans the desires of their hearts is to "take delight in him" and submit their will to his will.[15]

Method #3: Denying or Perverting the Truth in Scripture

Holy scripture is alive and active and contains truth that poses great danger to the enemy whose kingdom of darkness is built upon the foundation of lies.[16] Most religious faiths share the concern that their sacred writings may be misinterpreted or changed, giving our spiritual adversaries an advantage. For example, in Islam, there is a concept called *tahrif*, the belief that scriptures of previous revelations have been altered and thus corrupted and that the Quran is the sacred text sent to correct these distortions. Additionally, Hinduism teaches that misinterpretation of the Vedas or other sacred texts can lead to wrong practices, and Buddhism warns against wrong views (*miccha ditthi*) that distort the dharma.

As we discussed in Chapter 4, God's adversary successfully limited access to the written Bible for more than 1,400 years by several means. First, Scripture was under tight control of the hierarchical church in Rome, whose priests were the only ones authorized to teach from it. Second, for many years, Scripture was only translated into Latin, the language of the educated few, making it unavailable to the masses. Third, before Gutenberg invented the printing press in 1440, the few copies of Scripture were largely painstakingly copied by hand and valued so much they were typically chained to the pews at the local church.

A brave few saw the Bible as so important that they were willing to make the ultimate sacrifice of giving their lives in order to translate it into other languages or smuggle copies of translations in defiance of church law. Once new translations were made and copies were able to be reproduced more quickly following the invention of the printing press, the truth was out, and Satan needed a new strategy.

The Devil has successfully propagated the lie that the Bible is an irrelevant, outdated, boring book of rules without any historical basis or archaeological evidence, full of contradictions and inconsistencies, written by forty largely uneducated men. Probably the number one thought crime of today is the belief that the Bible is the inerrant Word of God. Satan blinds the spiritual eyes of unbelievers so they cannot see the "glorious light of the good news."[17]

The truth of the matter is that the Bible is an incredible Spirit-inspired narrative of sixty-six books written by forty authors over a nearly 1,500-year span, yet it has a consistent and coherent theological message from cover to cover. The accuracy of its predictive prophecy alone makes it stand apart from other sacred religious texts. Amazingly, the Bible we have today has been reliably handed down over the span of millennia, with only minor textual discrepancies. Despite numerous futile attempts over the centuries to ban the Bible or eradicate it altogether, it continues to be the best-selling book of all time.[18]

These attempts to deny or pervert the truth of Scripture are as old as the Garden of Eden:

But the Lord God warned him [Adam], "You may freely eat the fruit of every tree in the garden—except the tree of the knowledge of good and evil. If you eat its fruit, you are sure to die."[19]

One day he [the serpent] asked the woman, "Did God really say you must not eat the fruit from any of the trees in the garden."[20]

Satan questioned Eve's understanding of God's Word and in so doing, he expressed disbelief that God would say this, thus subtly drawing God's character into question. Then came Satan's next tactic. He proceeded to very slightly, but very importantly, twist God's Word, implying that the Creator was too restrictive in saying they could not eat the fruit from *any* of the trees. The truth is that God said they could eat from every tree except one. This is hardly restrictive.

What transpired next is of the utmost importance for us to recognize. When Eve repeated back God's Word to the nachash, she showed that she did not know it verbatim by the fact that she added to what God had said. According to Eve, not only were they forbidden to eat the fruit, but now they supposedly could not even touch it without dying. Seeing that he had drawn her in, Satan capitalized on her lack of orthodoxy by putting forth his biggest and boldest lie: "You won't die!" Satan insisted. He then returned to questioning God's goodness and his motives, again suggesting that he was restrictive, because God allegedly did not want mankind to become wise like him. Likely swayed by his beauty, wisdom, and superior knowledge of God and his Word, Eve gave way to the lust of the flesh (its fruit looked delicious), the lust of the eyes (the tree was beautiful), and the pride of life (she wanted the wisdom it would give her)—"She took some of the fruit and ate it."[21]

Method #4: Distraction from Spiritual Pursuits

There is a universal challenge to spiritual focus across all religious faiths. In Islam, the concept of *ghaflah* (heedlessness) describes being distracted by worldly matters, leading to neglect of religious obligations and hindering the connection to God. Hinduism speaks of the distractions of the senses and the mind that prevent focus on spiritual goals, while Buddhism identifies attachment to worldly pleasures as a hindrance to enlightenment.

Satan uses a multitude of distractions to keep slaves from seeking spiritual matters and finding the truth, but I will briefly discuss three of the most common tactics he employs today.

Busyness

The first distraction is busyness. While the internet, technology, and mobile devices have delivered on some of their promises to make people more productive, there are formerly hidden costs that are only now being reluctantly recognized. Physician, author, and educator Richard Swenson has written that progress has misled us into relying on it, only to drain us through an overwhelming array of choices and activities.[22] The intoxication of unlimited information and entertainment within our reach at all times, and in nearly all places, has turned technology into our culture's acceptable addiction.

As a child psychiatrist, I have witnessed firsthand the alarming shift in our culture to define progress for our children as "more." Compared to my generation's childhood, in the 1970s and 1980s, kids today seemingly have more of everything—more homework, more practices for sports, more entertainment options, and more toys, to name just a few. But there are also many more child and adolescent mental illnesses, and I can't help but think there is likely a correlation. Technology, social media, and gaming, for example, are not inherently bad. But as with anything else that can be addictive, we need to put guardrails around these to protect our children, both as parents and as a society. As the old saying goes, too much of a good thing can become a bad thing. Acceptable or not, media and electronic devices need to be increasingly recognized for what they are—addictive distractions that carry the same risks of enslavement that other addictions, such as substance abuse and gambling, do.

Busyness has squeezed our time, leaving little to no margin for us to deal with unexpected events that inevitably occur or to regularly engage in necessary self-care activities like physical exercise, spiritual practices, hobbies, rest and relaxation, and socialization. Because progress has very rapidly given us more and more, there are more options, opportunities, and obligations today, making it essential that we practice saying no to good things in order to lead a balanced life that will promote our physical, mental, and spiritual well-being. I agree with Dr. Swenson that people must be intentional and disciplined to restore a greater margin so that they are available for God's purposes. The fact is that the Devil has set up his kingdom with so many enticing and potentially addictive distractions that when God attempts to call the slaves to a new life of freedom, he gets a busy signal.

Pleasure

Pleasure is another effective distraction Satan uses, and I will address it further in the following section. In short, Satan has built a world system that exploits mankind's neurological makeup to reinforce pleasure-seeking behaviors. This leaves humans frustrated that they are unable to achieve the highs they seek and increasingly addicted to the things Satan's system offers as enticing alternatives to spiritual life.

Divisions

The final tactic Satan uses to discourage humans from spiritual pursuits is the manufacture of division. He knows well that a divided citizenry is much easier to control than a unified one. First, he sows division among organized religions. Even if his enslaved citizens desire to seek truth through organized religion, which one should they pursue? Hostility between Hindus, Muslims, Jews, and Christians becomes a barrier to truth seekers. Then, there are the multiple factions within each religion, such as Islam (with its multiple sects, schools, and branches), Judaism (with its four main branches of Orthodox, Reform, Conservative, and Reconstructionist), and Christianity (with its multiple denominations following fundamentally disparate doctrines), which make the prospect all the more confusing to slaves whose minds are already blinded to the truth. I have heard many people over the years express discouragement and confusion over the fact that different denominations all call themselves Christian yet believe very different things. If Christianity is the truth, they ask, why can't they all agree or at least get along?

More recent divisions along political and racial lines may also have a sinister, hidden force behind them. Most people would agree that they have never before seen the degree of discord that currently exists between political parties in the United States and also in other places around the world. There no longer seems to be a moderate middle ground, only polar opposite right- and left-wing factions, both of whom tend to demonize their opponents. Likewise, many believe that racial divisions are higher now than at any time in history, even than during the Civil Rights Movement of the 1960s. I believe this is satanic simply because God loves all people and commands his human children to love one another. Racism is evil because God says it is; he promises that one day people from every tribe, nation, and race will live in harmony in heaven, gathering around the throne to worship their God.[23] I pray that God's will regarding harmony among the races be done on earth as it will be in heaven.

Method #5: Debase Mankind and Exalt Physical Senses and Emotions

As the destroyer and the author of confusion, the Devil desires to undo God's created order. Having already cast doubt on the veracity and relevance of Scripture, the next logical step was for him to call into question creation itself. His lie, believed by many in the modern world today, is that there may be a God, but he is distant and uncaring. Hence, the physical universe in which we live came about by a Big Bang that had no first cause, and life evolved by random chance over many billions of years. There certainly was no garden with man created from dirt and woman created from one of man's ribs. And how absurd it is to believe that there was a talking snake who led them to sin. Humans are merely highly evolved animals who are the product of random chance, not tripartite beings created by God in his own image. This fairy tale was simply primitive, uneducated mankind's attempt to understand the scary world in which he found himself. That's the story the enemy continues to spin.

When Scripture describes how difficult it is for rich persons to escape the kingdom of darkness into which they were born and enter God's Kingdom of Light, I believe it is not only speaking of monetary riches, because there are relatively few in life who are actually rich in this way. There are riches of other kinds that people commonly possess, such as knowledge, social status, physical beauty, intelligence, talents, strength, and the like. There are many slaves who blindly travel through life on this broad road in which they place their trust in one or more of these riches. In today's modern world, one of the riches most often employed by Satan is knowledge.

Our adversary encourages the dismissal of religious truths as mere superstitions or outdated myths by promoting *scientism*, the belief that science is the ultimate path to knowledge, eclipsing other ways of understanding reality, such as theology. However, Scripture warns that knowledge on its own only puffs up a person, leading to intellectual arrogance, and that the very foundation of knowledge begins with reverence of God.[24]

The English word *science* has evolved over time and is derived from the Latin *scientia*, which originally meant knowledge in general and not just the field of natural sciences that employ methodology reliant on generating and testing hypotheses and then examining empirical evidence. Without question, the fields of natural science have contributed to the advancement of human knowledge and the betterment of society by providing explanations for natural phenomena, improving healthcare, and leading to technological advances. Although science has a provisional nature due to its hypotheses and theories being subject to change with new evidence, as contrasted with the absolute nature of spiritual truth, Satan has still successfully used it to influence modern mankind to question the reliability of faith-based knowledge that is not subject to the same methods of testing. Thus, Satan has used this as an opportunity to effectively employ the field of modern science as a means to sow doubt and lead people away from spiritual truth. The only valid and reliable kind of evidence according to Satan comes from testing things in the physical, material universe.

Spiritual practitioners of all religions, on the other hand, subscribe to the fundamental, unchanging belief in the existence of the divine and the authority of their holy scriptures that are not subject to the same empirical scrutiny used in the field of science. This is because science only addresses the "how" of the natural world, whereas theology addresses the "why" of existence and moral purpose. Scientific knowledge has essentially become the new religion to many modern people who place their faith in its tenets, which are subject to change. If you don't believe me, simply peruse any science book written before 1950 and you will see the evidence for yourself that scientific understanding changes dramatically over time with new discoveries.

Satan's next lie to his blinded and enslaved citizens of the kingdom of darkness is that since humans are merely highly evolved animals who are the product of random chance, life has no higher meaning or purpose other than to gratify one's physical senses. Morals are considered a social construct to control behavioral excesses rather than innate and objective obligations to the one who ultimately defines right and wrong. Thus, Satan has developed a world system that encourages moral relativity and materialism to gratify the physical senses and that not only discourages spirituality but openly mocks or even oppresses those who follow this path. This is evident by the fact that our culture regularly promotes entertainment, the acquisition of wealth and power, consumerism, alcohol and drug use, sexual promiscuity and perversion, gaming, social media, and the goals of leisure activities and early retirement over pursuing the meaningful, eternal work God desires.

Satan designed his world system to provide humans with more of the neurotransmitter responsible for pleasurable sensations: dopamine. But it turns out that endless dopamine hits do not satisfy. Instead, they leave the recipient always wanting more. This is the biological mechanism of all addiction, and the enemy uses it to further enslave his unwitting victims.

While emotions, such as pleasure, are not bad in and of themselves, they are the shallowest part of our being, as humans. Therefore, I routinely counsel patients not to allow their emotions to be the driving force in their life. Life has its ups and downs, and it is perfectly normal to prefer pleasure over more negative emotions, but the truth of the matter is that humans cannot continually live in a state of emotional highs. The primary reinforcing pattern of any addiction is that once people experience the pleasurable high, they erroneously believe Satan's lie that they should be allowed to live in that state, and therefore become enslaved to constantly seeking it.

Interestingly, neuroscience has more recently proven that humans were not designed to live in a persistently high-pleasure state. The nucleus accumbens (NAc), a subcortical component of the forebrain, plays a critical role in mediating reward, motivation, and emotions by receiving dopaminergic projections from a midbrain region called the ventral tegmental area (VTA). By means of this pathway, dopamine is released from the VTA to synapses in the NAc, where it assigns motivational salience to stimuli, such as food, sex, socialization, or drugs of abuse. Activation of the NAc drives behavior toward further exposure to the stimuli that led to the pleasurable sensation. But there is a neurological caveat to this system—repeated exposure to the same stimulus can result in neuroadaptive changes, such as reduced dopamine receptor sensitivity or dopamine release, both of which dampen the initial pleasurable response. This is likely the reason that drug and alcohol addicts tend to use increasingly larger amounts of their substance of choice in a futile attempt to recapture that initial pleasurable sensation they experienced when first using the substance, a phenomenon referred to as "chasing the dragon."

A final tactic Satan uses to debase mankind and keep us enslaved is sowing seeds of discontent about the way we were created. If human beings are simply the product of chance and evolution, then it would be reasonable to consider changing aspects of their being with which they are uncomfortable, such as their gender. However, if human beings are created by God in his image, it is a direct affront to their Creator to desire to change the way he created them. I believe that this very tangible example of mankind's self-will being exalted over God's will is a plot hatched by our invisible enemies. I see many children (and some adults as well) who are confused about their gender identity and have a strong desire to change their biological nature due to the associated intense dysphoria. While I genuinely empathize with their emotional distress, I generally encourage patients to first move toward acceptance of their biological fate in psychotherapy before considering radically attempting to change it through medical or surgical means. In my professional opinion, this stance is of utmost importance in children under the age of eighteen, who are, by nature, still developing and ethically should not be allowed to make a major medical decision that could possibly forever alter their biology and impair their ability to conceive children in the future.

I have observed a proliferation of severe mental illness among patients with gender dysphoria and confusion. This phenomenon was much rarer at the beginning of my career, in the 1990s, but it has exploded over the last decade. Compared to the rest of the population, transgender people are three to six times as likely to be autistic, according to the largest study yet to examine the connection.[25] Knowing that Satan hates God and his created human family, I find it plausible that he is the author of this confusion in an attempt to destroy the family, the God-ordained fundamental unit of human society. And it would be just like Satan, the lion seeking young vulnerable victims to devour, to sow gender confusion among innocent autistic children with inherent social problems. As the creator of the family, God has the absolute right to define its boundaries, which he decreed to be the union of one man and one woman, who would bring forth children to fill the earth by means of procreation.

From Slaves to Fear to Seekers of Freedom

According to the Judeo-Christian Bible, slavery is much more pervasive than a single individual or even an entire nation. All of mankind is under bondage since our spiritual adversary launched sin and death into the world. And with this, something else happened—the "fear of death" was born, a fear that subjected everyone to "slavery all their lives."[26] All of mankind is a slave to sin and fear, toiling our entire lives in shackles until the day our death sentence is finally carried out.[27] If you are one of the slaves whose mind has been so blinded by mankind's adversary that you believe humans exist briefly in this life on earth because of chance and evolution and that there is no God and no afterlife, then according to Scripture, you "are of all people most miserable and to be pitied."[28] The good news is that God loves mankind so much that he sent a deliverer to free us all from enslavement to sin and death.[29]

Satan capitalizes on mankind's innate fear of death by stealing one last thing—hope. In the 2012 dystopian motion picture *The Hunger Games*, the evil President Snow states the purpose of having a winner of the games is to control the people in the districts by giving them hope. "It is the only thing stronger than fear," he says. "A little hope is effective; a lot of hope is dangerous. A spark is fine, as long as it's contained."[30]

Satan would rather steal all hope so that his enslaved subjects will not even entertain any futile thoughts of future freedom. After all, small sparks can start big fires.

Enslaved citizens of the kingdom of darkness have no hope beyond the grave, making the prospect of death completely paralyzing to them. People are rightly terrified about death, and that's one reason why so many today are preoccupied with fear. The world system and media that Satan controls have done a masterful job of convincing the enslaved citizenry that the world is a very precarious and dangerous place. And Satan knows well that if he can magnify the potential of death by convincing people there is a looming threat, such as a terrorist attack or a pandemic that's going to kill them, then he can get them to do almost anything, without reason or purpose. They will even gladly give up their rights for perceived security. But the worst thing is not to live in this brief life as a slave without hope; it's to end up in the next life without hope forever.

Most enslaved citizens are surprisingly content to pursue pleasure and avoid the responsibility required to attain true freedom. As they develop, some people, especially those who actively pursue responsibility, have a rising sense of discontent, a feeling that things are not as they should be. These individuals come to realize they are slaves, and although they long to be free, they don't know how to achieve it, because the systems in place in the world are very powerful and designed to reinforce pleasure-seeking. These people observe that there are also a few foreigners living in their kingdom who seem to be free, despite the fact they are living under the same oppressive regime.

These foreigners possess a degree of peace and joy despite their circumstances, and they live a life characterized by love of others, sacrifice, and submission. They claim to be citizens of another kingdom whose ruler is a man who purposefully sacrificed his life thousands of years ago to somehow set them free from sin. They believe that their risen King will return one day to deliver his people physically and take over the world, becoming its one rightful ruler.

Most of these foreigners are easily dismissed because they claim to be different, but in reality, they live no differently from citizens of the kingdom of darkness. While these self-identified citizens of the Kingdom of Light claim to be free from the slavery of sin, many of them still sin just the same and tend to watch and listen to the same things, eat and drink the same things, and go to the same places as citizens of the kingdom of darkness do. While the majority of the foreigners seem to be counterfeits of something that is real and true, there is something unmistakably different about the very small subset of them who seem to genuinely follow the ruler of their foreign kingdom, the one who promises to destroy mankind's last enemy—death itself.[31]

Fortunately, some natural-born citizens of this seized kingdom of darkness retain a glimmer of hope and see a beckoning light shining in the darkness. Could there still be a chance of deliverance and freedom? The next chapter tackles that question.

10

STRATEGIC INTEL PART II: THE BATTLE PLAN FOR THE FREED SLAVES

We can easily forgive a child who is afraid of the dark;
the real tragedy of life is when men are afraid of the light.

—PLATO

The previous chapter described how the account of the enslaved Israelites' exodus from Egypt around 1446 BC provides a template of the four stages of life's spiritual journey, including a detailed description of the first phase—slavery. This chapter will explore Satan's strategies in the final three phases of mankind's spiritual journey: deliverance, wandering, and entrance into the Promised Land.

Phase 2 of the Spiritual Journey: Deliverance

The world's major religious faiths share the concept of liberation exemplified in the second phase of the spiritual journey. For example, in Islam, deliverance is achieved through submission to Allah and adherence to the Quran. Hinduism describes moksha, liberation from the cycle of rebirth, while Buddhism offers nirvana, freedom from suffering through enlightenment.

For Jews and Christians, Egypt and its enslavement of the Israelites represent the dwelling place of lost people under the control of lesser "gods," where there is idolatry and an emphasis on possessions, status, and sensuality. Egypt serves as a metaphor for the world system run by Satan, from which God's people need to be liberated. Fortunately, the Bible recounts that the people of Israel were miraculously delivered from their enslavement, just as everyone today who is enslaved by sin and Satan's rule can be.

The Jewish patriarch Abraham's grandson, whose name was changed to Israel after he wrestled with the angel of the Lord, had twelve sons whose descendants became the people of the nation named after him. One of Israel's sons, Joseph, was sold into slavery in Egypt by his brothers because they were jealous that Joseph was their father's favorite son. But what they intended to be evil, God turned to good, as Joseph successfully suffered through many trials and eventually rose from the rank of slave to the second-in-command in all of Egypt, behind only the pharaoh himself.[1]

When a famine arose in that part of the world, Israel and all of his family settled in Egypt, because the country had a plentiful supply of grain, due to Joseph's wise administration, and they were given protection under Joseph's supervision. The descendants of Israel multiplied over several hundred years in that land, and eventually, a pharaoh arose who, Scripture says, "knew not Joseph."[2]

The children of Israel were then collectively enslaved by the Egyptians, who perceived the Israelites to be a threat due to their growing numbers. The Israelites suffered bondage in Egypt for more than 400 years. Islam, Judaism, and Christianity all believe that God then sent a deliverer, the patriarch Moses. While there is no single deliverer in Hinduism and Buddhism, there are spiritual teachers—gurus or *bodhisattvas*—who play a vital role in guiding seekers toward liberation.

Because they were born into slavery, at some point the enslaved Israelites simply accepted their lot in life, just as today, most of the slaves born into Satan's kingdom of darkness also seem to have accepted their lot. They appear to be relatively content, likely because they have all their basic needs met and are not physically whipped or enchained. However, some experience a growing sense that things are not as they should be.

Just as God sent Moses to be the deliverer of the nation of Israel years before, God later sent his Messiah to earth to deliver the entire human family he loves. God calls all humans to accept the Messiah's sacrifice as payment for their sin debt, beckoning them out of the kingdom of darkness and into his marvelous light.[3]

Some born slaves see the light piercing through the darkness, emanating from the faithful foreign citizens of the Kingdom of Light. Some of these born slaves bravely respond to the beckoning of the light and achieve their freedom by accepting the pardon and pledging allegiance to the foreign King, thereby transferring their citizenship to the Kingdom of Light.[4]

This emancipation occurs when individuals come to their spiritual senses by responding to their Creator, earnestly seeking the higher power who first sought them, and turning their will and their lives over to God.[5] By means of his own death and resurrection, Jesus Christ legally took back the title deed to the earth forfeited by Adam and Eve and bought back all born slaves who willingly accept his sacrifice as payment for their sin debt.

Not only do these former slaves gain freedom and new citizenship, but amazingly, God himself adopts them as his children, making them legal heirs to his vast spiritual riches.[6] According to Christians, when Jesus returned to heaven after his mission was completed, he then established embassies in the occupied territory, called churches, which he staffed with ambassadors tasked with performing the ministry of reconciliation.[7] Until his promised return, the Messiah has granted God's adopted children authority to go into the entire world, delivering to anyone who will listen the good news of God's plan to reconcile each member of his human family with God.[8]

But to be delivered from the slavery into which they were unwittingly born, people must willingly accept the pardon God freely grants them. It is entirely possible to believe in God but reject the pardon and subsequent freedom he offers. The story of George Wilson is reminiscent of how some treat God's gracious offer.

In 1830, George Wilson was found guilty of six charges after he and another man robbed a mail carrier and jeopardized the carrier's life. Both men were sentenced to death, and Wilson's partner in crime was hanged later that year. But Wilson had influential friends, who petitioned the president of the United States, Andrew Jackson, for a pardon. President Jackson did, in fact, issue Wilson a full pardon, dropping all charges. Incredibly, Wilson refused to accept the pardon, and his case made it all the way to the US Supreme Court. Chief Justice John Marshall wrote the following in his opinion:

> *A pardon is an act of grace, proceeding from the power entrusted with the execution of laws. . . . [But] delivery is not complete without acceptance. It may then be rejected by the person to whom it is tendered, and . . . we have discovered no power in a court to force it on him.*[9]

George Wilson was subsequently executed. *What a fool!* many people today might think, without realizing that they, too, may be refusing a pardon—one that would enable them to be freed from spiritual bondage and spend eternity in the presence of God rather than being eternally separated from him in hell.

Deliverance from this slavery is a rescue mission with three stages: 1) deliverance from the penalty of sin, 2) deliverance from the power of sin, and then 3) deliverance from the very presence of sin. If someone accepts God's gracious gift of a pardon, the first stage of deliverance from the death penalty of sin is completed once and for all, as they are instantaneously made to be in legal right standing with God. Just as the ancient Israelite slaves were told to trust in the blood of an unblemished lamb painted on the doorposts of their homes to protect them from the angel of death on the night of Passover, people must put their trust in the atoning blood of the Lamb of God, Jesus, to save themselves from sin and death. The act of adoption into God's family and transfer of legal citizenship from the kingdom of darkness into his Kingdom of marvelous Light is made official.

But once a slave is pardoned, God doesn't remove them from the spiritual battle they were born into. God simply removes the bondage that certified allegiance to Satan.

The theological principle of "already, but not yet" is the reason that people, and especially newly freed citizens of the Kingdom of Light, still have a battle on their hands despite Jesus's victory over sin and death on the cross. Although God has put all things in subjection under Jesus, Scripture says, "We do not yet see all things put under him."[10]

Satan still has squatter's rights to the earthly domain to which he was cast.[11] And he is ferociously defending his territory because he knows full well that his time is short.[12]

Christians believe that when Jesus returns to earth with its title deed, he will judge Satan and the citizens of his kingdom of darkness who have not turned to God for their pardon. God will then take back control of the entire earthly kingdom that is rightfully his.

Until then, freed slaves must realize that their newfound freedom is not one without limits and guardrails. It is not a freedom from responsibility but rather a freedom to accept responsibility—to both God and fellow human imagers of him. No longer are freed slaves bound by the law of the jungle that was preeminent in the kingdom of darkness. As new citizens of the Kingdom of Light, they are now bound by a new set of laws predicated, according to Scripture, upon these two foundational laws: "You must love the Lord your God with all your heart, all your soul, all your mind, and all your strength . . ." and "Love your neighbor as yourself."[13]

Escaping the difficulties inherent in this fallen world by seeking pleasure, artificial substance-induced highs, or distractions through entertainment or gaming are no longer tenable solutions. The new rules no longer require humans to win at all costs, but they do demand that humans have the courage and perseverance to obey their new King's perfect law of freedom and never give up.[14] In this way, new citizens of the Kingdom of Light are more than citizens; they are also soldiers who can be trained to fight in the cosmic spiritual battle.

No longer nameless slaves, those who are freed become aware that they are unique and loved creations of their higher power with a responsibility to fulfill a personalized task in life. This fact enables them to overcome or endure difficulties and suffering, giving life significant meaning up until the final breath.[15]

Phase 3 of the Spiritual Journey: Wandering

Pardoned people are immediately imbued with power to act in accordance with God's purposes in their lives through his Spirit, which now dwells in them. But a person's day-to-day effectiveness against Satan's strategies is still a matter of submission—a freed person can still submit to either God's will or their own.

This is why newly freed slaves enter into the next phase of their spiritual journey, in which they are enlisted in the infantry and move from civilian life to military life. Now that they are awakened to the reality of a spiritual war being waged by powerful unseen enemies, freed slaves must now relinquish expectations of ease and comfort and fully embrace the reality that they are at war.

While there is a legitimate training experience for this phase of one's spiritual journey, Christianity and Judaism believe a lack of spiritual discipline or a continued attachment to the charms of the world will prolong time in the training wilderness.[16] This was the case for the ancient Israelites freed from Egypt, whose journey to the Promised Land should have taken fourteen days. Instead, it lasted forty years due to their stubbornness and rebellion.

Before becoming combat ready, newly enlisted soldiers must go through several stages of training. The first stage of training involves former slaves recovering from the wounds of their past. Because the only way to reach the Promised Land is through this military training in the proverbial wilderness, the next stage of training involves a laborious time of trials in which newly enlisted soldiers of the Kingdom of Light have the opportunity to either become promoted to the status of officer through the progressive process of sanctification or to remain stagnant in their rank and journey.

God actually sends or allows adversity to test the character, faith, and holiness of his adopted children.[17] Such tests involve difficult external circumstances that people are led into by the Spirit of God in order to assess the degree of their faith. These can range from mere setbacks in one's plans to experiencing financial difficulties, not having one's needs met, or suffering persecution, injustice, disease, or death, to name a few. The belief that challenges refine the soul is also seen in Hinduism, where *tapas* (austerity) purifies the soul through hardship, and in Buddhism, which teaches the Middle Way to balance extremes on the spiritual path.

New soldiers must strive to pass their tests by keeping them external and relying upon their higher power. When God's children fail and internalize their tests, these trials become an open door that Satan utilizes to lie to them, entice them to respond in a manner contrary to God's will, and build strongholds in their minds.

There are several important purposes behind this time of training for newly freed slaves. First, God uses trials to train people to grow stronger and more useful to him and to help accomplish his kingdom objectives.[18] God sometimes employs trials of physical pain, medical conditions, or illness to keep people humble and reliant on him, as he did in the life of the Apostle Paul, who "was given a thorn in [his] flesh, a messenger from Satan to torment [him] and keep [him] from becoming proud."[19] Apparently, despite his pleadings and fervent prayer, God never did take away Paul's ailment. And Paul not only accepted his suffering ordained by God but was also able to boast about it, recognizing that, as the Scripture says, God's "power works best in weakness."[20]

In Christianity, God also employs trials to wean patients from worldly things, training them to long for the true treasures of heaven and to "suffer with the people of God rather than enjoy the fleeting pleasure of sin."[21] Likewise, Hinduism and Buddhism view suffering as a tool to detach from worldly desires and gain spiritual insight.

Finally, God uses trials in people's lives to enable them to help others who are suffering.

While God, in his love for us, employs trials to better prepare his soldiers for his purposes in their lives and others', Satan employs a counterattack against anyone who has turned his or her back on his kingdom. It is therefore critical to know the difference between a training exercise from God and an attack from the enemy. As we've previously discussed, the primary way to know the authentic from the counterfeit is to know the authentic thing so well you can always spot what is false. The same is true when it comes to knowing whether an adverse circumstance is training or an outright attack. But either way, God's children have the assurance that he will use any event in our lives for the good of his kingdom.[22]

Satan's Tactics for Freed Slaves in the Wilderness of Training

Chapter 3 took an in-depth look at Satan's global plans in the past, present, and future. The remainder of this chapter will focus on his plans against individual human beings. After all, his best opportunity to retaliate against God is to hinder and harm his children—those God has bought out of slavery.

Physical, Psychological, and Spiritual Hindrances

Satan attempts to hinder and harm God's freed slaves physically (through sickness, other people, animals, weather, etc.), psychologically (through lying messages, bitterness, slander, fear, etc.), and spiritually (through misplaced worldly priorities, infiltration of the church, hindering one's ministry, service, or witness).

Just as we should anticipate problems on a national or global level due to satanic influence in the world as a whole, the same holds true for adversity in our personal lives. As difficult as it may be to fathom, God decreed plans and purposes for each individual's life before they were ever conceived, and he promises to work all things, even suffering and adverse circumstances, together for good.[23] While it is true that adversity happens in life, more often than not, there is a hidden hand orchestrating much of it and attempting to thwart God's purposes and plans.

Make no mistake: If people are living according to God's will and plans for their lives, they will be attacked by their unseen spiritual enemies. These enemies know God's plans—not only for mankind over vast periods of time in human history (albeit not completely) but also for individual members of his family—and they aim to hinder those plans and harm God's family in the process.

From Suppressing the Truth to Hindering Belief

Satan is a murderer at his core, whose last countermove in the spiritual war nearly 2,000 years ago was to influence his sons of disobedience to kill God's redeemer on a Roman cross once he was revealed to the world. Because Jesus's glory was veiled in human flesh, Satan and his demonic horde likely did not initially realize that Jesus came to die as a sacrifice to pay the sin debt of all mankind throughout history.

Fooled, resoundingly defeated, and stripped of his authority following Jesus's crucifixion and resurrection, Satan's strategy turned to hindering the good news of God's pardon from getting out in the first place by building his kingdom of darkness upon a foundation of lies and control of his enslaved populous. But once the good news became widely known anyway, Satan pivoted again by attempting to prevent people from believing it, a strategy that has proven to be relatively successful over the past 2,000 years.

Today, Satan operates behind the scenes to attempt to kill humans by influencing them to become self-destructive by means of suicide, addiction to alcohol or drugs, or a sexually immoral lifestyle. I believe he especially likes these methods because they allow him to keep his hands clean, essentially allowing people themselves to do his dirty work to thwart God's good plans for their lives. While Satan is not permitted to directly kill children of God, he can attempt to bring about their deaths by means of other people, weather and natural disasters, accidents, animals, and sickness, to name a few. According to Scriptural examples, the general principle is the greater Satan's attack, the greater God's plans for the individual.

Hindering God's Purposes in Believers' Lives

Another common strategy of the enemy is to prevent, hinder, or at least delay God's purposes in the lives of his children. Although his freed slaves have been emancipated and Satan can no longer hope to keep them from God and take them to hell with him, Satan can and does hinder their ministry, service, and witness by wounding them, defiling them, and attempting to make them bitter against people or institutions who have harmed them.

When they were slaves living in the kingdom of darkness, they were not even aware that they were involved in a spiritual war. So, it is not surprising that former slaves have unwittingly accumulated heart wounds from their demonic foes over the course of their life by metaphorically walking through the battlefield of the world without any protection. But now that the spiritually awakened and freed slaves have been reconciled with God, the Great Physician and healer's Spirit gives them power, authority, and discernment to help fight the spiritual war.

Working through the steps of Ruachiatry, which I'll discuss in detail in Section III, can be an effective tool, enabling you to heal these wounds and subsequently don spiritual armor to protect yourself from getting re-wounded by Satan. Depending on the duration of time an individual has spent in slavery and the degree of trauma they have experienced, some may have deeper and more serious emotional wounds that require outside help from a psychotherapist.

As ruler over the kingdom of darkness, Satan has vast resources at his disposal to attack God's children, such as his hordes of demons, his enslaved "children of disobedience," and the entire world system with its many intricate branches, which he personally controls. The majority of the time, demonic attacks on God's freed slaves do not reach an extent that endangers their lives but rather propagate lies and build strongholds in their minds, to harass them and to sow discord. For example, believers' invisible enemies can motivate human subjects who are under the control of Satan to persecute the believers. The encounter I described in Chapter 8 with the man who inexplicably verbally berated me for the way I parked my car is an example of this in action. And I'm certain that every reader can think of instances in their own lives when they wondered if some unseen evil force might be behind the persecution or injustice they suffered.

Clearly, Satan can and does often use his unbelieving "children of disobedience" to harass, hinder, and even test believers. Faiths other than Christianity also give warnings about negative influences. Islam teaches that Shaytan tempts through others. Judaism warns of the Yetzer Hara's influence via societal pressures, and both Hinduism and Buddhism caution against those who are not on the spiritual path leading one astray.

Satan's Use of the World System

But the most common instrument the ruler of this world uses against believers is his vast world system. Life as soldiers fighting their former master Satan is indeed difficult. It involves courage and sacrifice, and it is paramount that they do not look back. They must resist temptations to return to their metaphoric enslavement.[24] This can be surprisingly challenging, because life is easier when one is not constantly engaged in battle.

Satan's world system includes many things that, by design, appeal to mankind's physical senses and emotions. Mankind's adversary has masterfully designed a world system that draws believers' focus to temporal, worldly things (not necessarily bad or sinful things) and away from eternal, spiritual pursuits. Satan desires to nullify the potential positive impact that God's soldiers can have on the world by promoting materialism, covetousness, lack of contentment, comparison with others, overloaded schedules without margin built in, and misplaced priorities.

Believers must be careful not to adopt misplaced priorities or get too comfortable in this brief life on earth because, Scripture warns, "friendship with the world makes you an enemy of God."[25] Jesus gave his followers "a gift the world cannot give . . . peace of mind and heart."[26] The enticing distractions Satan's world system offers will not ultimately satisfy; they are temporal and passing away.[27]

Furthermore, God's soldiers must resist the urge to have the best of both worlds, living with one foot in this world run by Satan and the other foot in God's kingdom. Once people are awakened to the fact they are involved in an invisible spiritual war, each individual must then choose a side. Neutrality in this war is not an option. Jesus made this clear when he said, "Whoever is not with me is against me."[28]

I once heard a story of a soldier who during the American Civil War wanted to improve his odds of survival. He hatched a plan to don a blue coat, like the Northern Army, and gray pants, like the Southern troops. Guess what happened?

He got shot from both sides!

Compromise can be deadly, and newly freed slaves must realize that wearing a patchwork spiritual uniform that is a blend of God's standards and the world's standards is not safe. You must choose sides wisely in this spiritual war and then be thoroughly and completely committed to your choice.

Exploiting Trials and Temptations

Probably Satan's most common and effective tactic is to take advantage of trials from God that are meant to test the faith of believers and further their spiritual development. By turning these into temptations to sin, Satan encourages believers to seek solace in a return to indulging their natural fleshly appetites via the world system. While many freed slaves are now equipped to see through his lies and former tactics, Satan is still often able to successfully deceive, distract, and divert believers' focus to sensuality and emotions, building mental strongholds that trap believers in some habitual sin, stunt their spiritual growth, and nullify the positive impact they have on others.

If freed slaves fall for Satan's temptation to exercise their spiritual liberty by dancing too close to the boundaries placed by God for their protection, they can easily fall back into sin and disqualify themselves as useful to God's service. This is the reason for the scriptural admonition: "Therefore let the one who thinks he stands firm, take care that he does not fall."[29]

It is important for freed slaves to understand that the inherited sin nature remains in their bodies until the promised future day when the final phase of God's redemption plan will be accomplished, and they will be given new eternal bodies without a sin nature, impervious to sickness and death itself. So, even though they now possess the Spirit's power over sin in the midst of their journey to the proverbial Promised Land, God's soldiers must be vigilant and disciplined to appropriate this power. No soldier in the Kingdom of Light will be sinless in this lifetime, but each one should progressively sin less than they used to.

Satan knows human nature well and therefore uses the same tactics again and again. For now, the Accuser is still allowed to prosecute his case against believers in front of the Judge, and according to Scripture, he does so with great vigor "day and night."[30] He relishes his role as patrolman of the earth, searching for opportunities to tempt God's children to stray, just as he did to God's faithful servant Job many years ago. Satan then prosecutes his case against them, suggesting that their faith is not genuine and that they actually do not love God but only the blessings he grants them. However, believers now have the very best defense attorney, a powerful advocate who, Scripture says, "lives forever to intercede with God on their behalf."[31] "So now there is no condemnation for those who belong to Christ Jesus," and the righteous Judge dismisses each case against his children, because "the power of the life-giving Spirit has freed [them] from the power of sin."[32]

False Teachers and Deceitful Workers to Create Counterfeit Believers

One final point about the tactics of this enemy: Perhaps his most sinister plot against God's soldiers is infiltrating God's church with false teachers, counterfeit believers, and deceitful workers, who disguise themselves as apostles of Christ.

We established earlier that Satan is a thief, but he is also a usurper, one who seizes and holds power and position without right. Since God created humans and also redeemed believers with the blood of his Messiah, God not only has legal right to ownership of those who trust him but also to ownership of the corporate body of them, called the church.

In biblical times, after the father of a bridegroom or the bridegroom himself paid a dowry to a bride or her parents, the betrothal period began. This was an extended length of time during which the bride and groom were separated before the wedding. In Scripture, Jesus is called the bridegroom and the church his bride, which waits during this betrothal period, called the "church age," for the bridegroom's return. At that time, the marriage ceremony will commence.[33] This bride and groom metaphor displays the degree of love, commitment, and covenant God desires in the relationship between him and his faithful church.

In Scripture, Jesus is also called the Good Shepherd, signifying his role as the spiritual head of the church, who is committed to knowing, feeding, leading, and protecting his flock.[34] Until his return, God has called certain soldiers to serve the church as *pastors*, a term that comes from the Greek word *poimen*, which translates to "shepherd."[35] Satan is described by Jesus himself as the thief who does not enter the sheep pen by the gate but by some other way, because he has sinister motives.[36] God's soldiers must develop discernment to realize that not everyone with a seminary degree who wears priestly robes and claims to follow God is a legitimate, Spirit–filled fellow soldier. Jesus taught that the true test of discernment in this matter is to closely observe the life of the person for evidence of fruit, or lack thereof, produced in their lives.[37] Satan influences ungodly persons, including pastors, to creep into churches stealthily and poison believers from within using disinformation.[38]

While misinformation refers to accidental untruth, disinformation is the intentional misrepresentation of the truth. False teachers within the church spread deceptive doctrines promulgated by the demonic forces influencing them, causing believers to fall away from the faith.[39] These false teachers preach another Jesus, another Spirit, and another gospel from the ones described in Scripture.[40]

Jesus himself warned his followers that during the end times, "many shall come in my name, saying, I am Christ, and shall deceive many."[41] False teachers influenced by Satan present an alternative Christ who is not the same person as the Jesus revealed in the Bible. For example, many mainstream Christian churches downplay the fact that Jesus himself claimed to be the Son of God, who came to offer himself as a sacrifice to reconcile mankind with God the Father. Many Christian churches today, and organizations like the one behind the "He Gets Us" television campaign, present a caricature of a hippie-like, all-loving Jesus who emphasized doing good works toward fellow men rather than practicing faith for salvation. These same groups often downplay what they consider to be the narrow-minded views that the Jesus of the Bible proclaimed, such as there is only one way to God and Jesus's demands for holiness and obedience in his followers. As C. S. Lewis pointed out, Jesus was either Lord, lunatic, or liar—his historical claims and well-documented life give us no other options.[42]

Several examples of "another" Jesus are the Mormon Jesus and the Jehovah's Witness Jesus. The Mormon Jesus is very different from the Jesus of Scripture in that followers believe there was nothing supernatural about his conception or birth and that Jesus is the literal spirit brother of Lucifer, the great angel who fell and became Satan. Jehovah's Witnesses believe that the Son of God was the archangel Michael before he came to earth, and John 1:1 in their version of the Bible states that Jesus was "a god."

False teachers within the church also present "another" Spirit, primarily through counterfeit power, signs, and wonders.[43] If this is not the Spirit of God, clearly it is a malevolent spirit working to deceive through sorcery (as in the case of Simon the sorcerer in the book of Acts), magic (as in the case of the Egyptian magicians mimicking the first four miracles that God worked through Moses), or supernatural events.[44]

Since power, signs, and wonders can be produced by both God and Satan, the Bible states that God's soldiers must "test the spirits" on their declaration of Jesus's identity to determine their source.[45] These soldiers must also resist the temptation to use their "natural" mind to discern the activity of God's Spirit and instead rely on the truth of Scripture, because the authentic Holy Spirit will never contradict Scripture.[46]

Jesus's last commandment to his followers was to "go into all the world and preach the gospel to every creature."[47] The gospel is the "good news" that Jesus paid for mankind's sins, providing an opportunity for every living person to be pardoned of their sin debt before God and be reconciled to him as adopted sons and daughters.

But in an attempt to see membership numbers increase, some false teachers today present "another gospel" that requires no understanding of sin, judgment, or atonement. The tragic consequence is that these teachings produce false converts who follow their own emotions as a guide to truth and erroneously believe they are in good standing with God. Churches that promote another gospel tend to be emotionally driven and entertainment focused, with services often looking more like the world system than the traditional church. An example of this is seen today in some megachurches, with false teachers who present a prosperity gospel that promises health and wealth to attract people who simply want to use God to improve their life situation. Satan's plan is to use these counterfeit, phony believers to confuse nonbelievers, minimize the impact God's soldiers could have on the world, and create discord and divisions within the body of believers itself.

Other faiths share Christianity's concerns about false believers. Islam warns of hypocrites (*munafiqun*) who undermine the faithful community. Judaism warns of false prophets, and both Hinduism and Buddhism caution against deceptive gurus or teachers who mislead followers.

Satan's infiltration into houses of worship serves the purpose of creating doubt in the minds of God's soldiers. Their enemy works hard to influence soldiers to doubt not only God's love but also Scripture itself. The idea that the Bible is a God-inspired, errorless book that is still relevant in the twenty-first century is either dismissed or ridiculed by most in our technologically advanced society. To the unbelieving slaves of Satan whose minds have been blinded by their master so that they cannot see the glorious light of the good news, the Word of God is a rock of offense.[48] In response, freed slaves are commanded to "preach the word . . . for the time will come when [some] will not tolerate sound doctrine; but wanting to have their ears tickled, they will accumulate for themselves teachers in accordance with their own desires, and they will turn their ears away from the truth and will turn aside to myths."[49]

It sure seems like we've already reached this time.

Soldiers in the midst of the battle must regularly remind themselves that biblical hope is a reality, not a feeling, that it is an assurance based on a secure, solid foundation, which their enemy wants to debunk. There is always hope, and the only certain and secure hope in a dangerous and rapidly changing world is in a loving, immutable God, who graciously offers salvation to his prodigal children.

Phase 4 of the Spiritual Journey: Storming the Promised Land

The final stage of deliverance that is promised in the future is deliverance from the very presence of sin, when God returns to purge the earth of its evil spiritual enemies and unrepentant human evildoers and reward believers with eternal glorified bodies that are incapable of sin. At this time, all disease, and even death itself, will be eradicated as all of creation will be made new. This aspiration for ultimate spiritual triumph is common to all faiths. In Islam, paradise (*Jannah*) offers eternal peace. Judaism anticipates the Messianic Age and *olam ha-ba* (world to come). Hinduism seeks moksha, freedom from rebirth, while Buddhism aims for nirvana, the end of suffering. According to Christianity, this blessed hope of ultimate redemption of all creation will only happen when the spiritual and human enemies occupying the Promised Land have been vanquished once and for all, enabling citizens of the Kingdom of Light to permanently settle there in peace, with God's Messiah reigning as king.

In the Biblical Exodus account, the Promised Land of Canaan is not only a picture of the future glory but also a picture of the victorious life of God's people despite enemies, giants, and other obstacles. They are, according to Scripture, "more than conquerors."[50] And, like Joshua, the Israelite military commander who led his people into the Promised Land after forty years of wandering in the wilderness, they are called to be strong in the power of the Lord and courageous because he is with them wherever they go.[51]

By demonstrating courage and perseverance during many trials in the wilderness, freed slaves will become soldiers who get promoted through the ranks to officer status and finally to special forces warriors by the time they reach God's Promised Land. By the power of God's Spirit and the Word of God, which is the Sword of the Spirit, these spiritual warriors will appropriate their God-given authority to take the land God has promised to his beloved adopted children.

11

BATTLEFIELD INTEL: THE MIND

The spiritual battle, the loss or victory, is always in the thought world.

—FRANCIS SCHAEFFER

In military operations, "battlefield intel" refers to terrain analysis, communications intercepts, and the critical intelligence about the enemy's size, positions, movements, armament, supply levels, morale, readiness, and psychological state, all of which can influence the timing and nature of attacks. It is vital for both planning defense strategies and coordinating attacks. In this chapter, we will discuss where the spiritual war is fought—the human mind.

Brain, Mind, Heart, and Spirit

We discussed earlier that humans are created as tripartite beings, composed of body, soul, and spirit. These three components interact with each other but have distinct functions. The body is the part that receives information from the physical world via the five senses and then is able to interact with the physical environment. The soul (*psyche* in Greek) is typically associated with the mind, emotions, will, and the very essence of individual identity that perceives the inner psychological world. Because the mind is part of our very soul, Satan much prefers to cripple it than the body. Experience shows that humans can accomplish incredible things with a crippled body and a sound mind (Stephen Hawking, for example), but a crippled mind tends to greatly hinder accomplishments, even if the body exhibits robust health.

The third component of human beings, the spirit, is universal to all faiths. Muslims, Jews, and Christians believe God's breath (*ruh* in Islam, *ruach* in Judaism) gives rise to the spirit that perceives the unseen spiritual world and enables humans to commune with and receive guidance from the divine. Hindus believe that the *atman* is the eternal spiritual core linked to Brahman, while Buddhists view consciousness (*viññāṇa*) as central to life.

Even though the soul and spirit are distinct, they are deeply interconnected.[1] The soul acts like a mediator between the physical body and the spirit. The ethereal portion of the soul, called the mind, enables humans to be conscious of both the physical and spiritual worlds and to think and feel. It is the actual battlefield where Satan and unclean spirits conduct their war against humanity.

The enemy knows that if he can control humans' thoughts, attention, and emotions, he can greatly influence their behavior, and perhaps their ultimate destiny as well. If we are to live holy lives pleasing to God, then mere conformity of our external behavior is not enough. As Scripture says, we must "first wash the inside . . . and then the outside will become clean, too."[2] The sum of our thoughts form our attitudes, which, in turn, lead to our actions. The late pastor Dr. Adrian Rogers succinctly summarized this process by reiterating Ralph Waldo Emerson's truism:

The thought is the father of the deed . . . "*Sow a thought, reap a deed. Sow a deed, reap a habit. Sow a habit, reap a character. Sow a character, reap a destiny.*"[3]

The mind processes information and then makes logical sense of it by formulating thoughts that eventually become actions. While the mind is the birthplace of thoughts, the "heart" (not the muscular organ that pumps blood, but the moral center) is associated with emotions, affections, conscience, and values. But the heart also functions to process the thoughts birthed by the mind, reflect on truth, and then make moral decisions. The concept of the heart as the core of spiritual faith and devotion is expressed in many faiths: *qalb* in Islam, *hridaya* in Hinduism, and *citta* in Buddhism, for example.

The heart is so important that the wise King Solomon of Israel advised his son nearly 3,000 years ago to "Guard your heart above all else, for it determines the course of your life," for as a man "thinks in his heart, so is he."[4] The people of the world judge by external standards, such as appearances, accomplishments, and position, but "the Lord looks at the heart," because he knows that what is inside will eventually be expressed outwardly.[5]

While the heart and mind are distinct, they work together, influencing each other in our decision-making, actions, and relationship with God. The thoughts from the mind can shape the emotions and desires of the heart, which in turn acts as a window between the spirit and the mind. The condition of our hearts influences how we think. A pure heart allows God's light to shine brightly on our minds, leading to godly reasoning. Conversely, a heart hardened by many years of unrepented sin may result in a mind that is closed or resistant to spiritual truths.[6] In the process of spiritual transformation, God renews both the heart and mind to align with his purposes.[7]

The heart of mankind is endowed with a conscience, a word derived from the Latin *conscientia*, which, when literally translated, means "with knowledge." C. S. Lewis believed the conscience is evidence for the existence of a moral law, a universal standard of right and wrong that all humans are born "with knowledge" of, even if they sometimes choose to disobey it.[8] This moral law cannot be fully explained as a social construct, a human invention, or a result of education or natural causes, and it suggests the existence of a higher power, a lawgiver who instills this law within all humans.[9] This innate moral compass is echoed in other faiths: *fitrah* in Islam, *Yetzer Tov* in Judaism, *dharma* in Hinduism, and *sila* in Buddhism.

This conscience serves to warn us when we're about to make a wrong choice or affirm us when we've made the right one. Just as the Creator equipped humans with the physical sensation of pain to warn us when there is some problem with our physical body, God gave us a conscience to warn us of spiritual problems.

In the absence of a spiritual rebirth, people often rack up years of unrepented sin, accumulating guilt in their conscience. The ongoing alarm offered by their conscience during this time can be silenced in various ways, with alcohol or drugs or by escape into relationships, fantasy, hobbies, pornography, sports, music, and entertainment. Since peoples' consciences will conform to the highest moral standard their soul perceives, it is of utmost importance that they thoughtfully and diligently work to identify whom they believe to be the Highest Power and then submit their will to his.

Analogy of a Computer System

I believe that the holistic system of the brain, mind, and spirit, where physical, mental, and spiritual components interact to form the complete human experience, is analogous to how hardware, software, and electrical power work together to make a computer function.

First, as the computer's hardware consists of circuits, processors, and memory that manage data processing and system operations, our brains are made up of neurons, synapses, and various physical structures that process information, control bodily functions, and enable the execution of tasks. Additionally, the brain stores memories, skills, and learned behaviors, much like a computer stores files and data in its hard drive or memory chips.

Second, the human mind is a control center for thoughts, emotions, consciousness, reasoning, and decision-making processes, analogous to the software or operating system that runs on a computer's hardware to operate it and execute specific tasks. Just as software provides the interface through which a user interacts with a computer, the mind is the interface through which we experience and interact with the world by interpreting sensory input, managing mental processes, and determining how to respond to our environment. The mind, like software, can be updated, changed, and influenced by experiences, learning, and external factors. It can adapt, develop new capabilities, and even "crash" under certain conditions, such as brain injury, neurological illness, or episodes of severe mental illness.

Lastly, the spirit in this analogy is the life force or divine essence that can be likened to the power source of the computer. Without this connection, both peoples' brains (the computer's hardware) and, to a greater extent, their minds (software) are markedly less effective, possibly even rendered useless for their created purpose. The spirit connects individuals to a transcendent higher power and to a sense of higher meaning and purpose beyond the material world, much like a network connection allows a computer to access information beyond its internal storage. Just as a computer requires a continuous power supply to function, the spirit can be seen as the sustaining life force that enables a deeper sense of vitality, direction, and connection to others and to the divine.

An optimally functioning computer requires all three elements—hardware, software, and electrical power—working together. Similarly, a human being functions optimally when the brain, mind, and spirit are in harmony. Just as software cannot operate without hardware and power, the mind cannot function without the brain's physical structures and the spirit's animating force.

When humans were slaves born into this physical world with a dead spirit due to their inherited sin nature, it was relatively easy for their powerful spiritual enemies to control their minds and their subsequent behavior, because without the spirit, the human mind is completely focused on the physical world and the drive to gratify the appetites of the physical body. These slaves lacked both the desire and the ability to live their life in the good and holy manner that their Creator originally intended. But this does not mean that human beings cannot do good things—it just means that, without a spirit, they do not desire to act altruistically without having ulterior motives, such as social approbation or other internal or external rewards.

But when some of the slaves miraculously experience a spiritual awakening and then believe and receive the pardon and path of healing offered by God, their dead spirit is made alive by God's own Spirit, giving them both the will and ability to live a holy lifestyle.[10] With this spiritual rebirth, people are no longer automatons reacting to the world in a selfish way to maximize their pleasure and minimize their pain; they are now free imagers of God, equipped to interpret the world and their relationship to it differently and to respond in a way their higher power desires.

To wrap up this imperfect yet useful analogy, Satan operates on the battlefield of the mind in a manner similar to computer viruses.

Viruses are analogous to demonic spirits in that they are malicious software that first gain entrance and then spread and cause damage to the computer's data, software, and systems. Viruses are designed to be stealthy and infect computers discreetly, and then to cripple computer performance, damage or destroy computer files, steal sensitive private information, and ultimately hijack control of the entire system.

Many today erroneously believe that the only thing wrong with the human mind is a lack of knowledge, that more education is the grand means of improving the human condition and fixing the world's problems. The issue is much deeper. No amount of education will eradicate selfishness, lying, stealing, killing, addiction, physical abuse, terrorist plots, or rape, because the problem is that people have fallen minds, software infected with the fatal virus of sin.

The condition of the human heart is just as grave, because it "is the most deceitful of all things and desperately wicked."[11] The heart of the human problem is the problem of the human heart. The longer people are enslaved in the kingdom of darkness, the more they are metaphorically exposed to viruses (spiritual enemies), without anti-malware (spiritual armor and God's Spirit) to protect them. These malevolent viruses invade, lay a foundation of lies, and then replicate the lies to erect a fortress within their victims' minds.

These are spiritual strongholds that can only be dismantled by spiritual means. Once people experience spiritual rebirth, their minds receive a powerful upgraded operating system, running on new software with antivirus protection the Bible calls "the mind of Christ."[12] Those who are spiritually reborn gain a new source of power and protection, the new Spirit, which acts to filter their experiences and thoughts. With this new power and protection, people must then be continually vigilant, guarding the gates of their minds through which their unseen enemies can still gain access.[13] They must also be sure to tear down the strongholds built by lies and to continually renew their minds with spiritual truths.[14]

Gates and Doors

In studying serial killers as part of my forensic psychiatry training, I recall learning about the case of Richard Trenton Chase, a serial killer known as the "Vampire of Sacramento." When the investigating FBI agent, Robert Ressler, asked Chase how he selected his victims, Chase chillingly replied that he simply walked the streets testing the doors of homes until he found one that was unlocked. He considered this to be an invitation, giving him the right to enter.

This is precisely how spiritual enemies operate—they look for open doors, unguarded minds. Before spiritual rebirth, the doors to peoples' minds were wide open and unguarded, allowing enemies unfettered access to build and then occupy mental fortresses based on a foundation of lies from the Devil that people believe to be true. Sin, trauma, fear, and anger can all act as those unlocked doors, giving malevolent forces a way in. Eastern traditions, such as Hinduism and Buddhism, add that ignorance and attachment also make people spiritually vulnerable. Open doors are how demonic foes gain entrance to peoples' minds, and strongholds are how they stay.

But just as these doors can be opened, they can also be closed.

The first step is learning the sins that commonly open doors in the first place. While demonic access to peoples' minds certainly includes sin in general, people must be aware of seven particular transgressions against God (three mental attitudes, three behaviors, and one circumstance outside of patients' control) that are well known to especially attract and empower malevolent entities.

Tolerance

The first common mental attitude that acts as an open door might surprise you. It is *tolerance*, a common buzzword today that has the connotation of virtuous open-mindedness and acceptance of the beliefs and behaviors of others with whom we disagree. But tolerance of beliefs or behaviors that violate God's standards is a sinister, slippery slope leading invariably to gradual moral decay within a society. Once again, the Devil's tactic is to amplify mankind's freedom while minimizing the inherent responsibility to God and fellow humans that such freedom carries. Today's popular biblical mantra of "judge not, that you be not judged" does not mean humans have no right to pronounce a value judgment on the beliefs or behaviors of other humans. On the contrary, the quote in its full context means spiritually reborn humans are to use their renewed minds to exercise discernment and to only employ God's standards in their judgments. But make no mistake, Scripture clearly states believers are indeed supposed to judge, just not in a hypocritical fashion in which they employ a different, more permissive standard for themselves.[15]

Tolerance is a means by which demonic influence enters a society, but these clandestine foes remain by shifting to intolerance once they are entrenched in power. Jesus himself chastised the first-century church in Thyatira—modern-day Turkey—for tolerating the spirit that had influenced Israel's wicked Queen Jezebel nearly 900 years prior; apparently, this same spirit was working through a false prophetess in Thyatira who was leading believers into a lifestyle of immorality.[16] Tolerance of the wrong things can be destructive or even deadly.

Fear and Uncontrolled Anger

The other two common mental attitudes known to be open doors to demonic influence are *fear*, which leads to a state of anxiety, and *uncontrolled anger*, which leads to resentment and bitterness. I'll discuss these fully in Chapter 14, specifically regarding Steps 5 and 8 of the proposed 12 Steps of Ruachiatry.

Traumas

Traumas that people experience are the most common circumstances outside their control that serve as open doors. Traumas are the number one means by which demonic foes are able to successfully deliver lies that become the foundation of mental strongholds in believers and nonbelievers alike. Traumas will also be discussed more fully in Chapter 14, specifically in Step 4.

In my nearly three-decade career as a psychiatrist, the two most common behaviors I have witnessed that open doors to spiritual enemies are *substance abuse* and *dabbling in occult practices*.

Substance Abuse

Patients under the influence of hallucinogenic drugs—such as LSD, psilocybin, DMT, ayahuasca, ketamine, nitrous oxide, and PCP— experience a sense of detachment from the physical world and also have "trips" that often have a spiritual component.

It is my professional opinion that the "trips" people experience and the entities they encounter while under the influence of hallucinogens cannot always be explained as merely the product of dopamine-induced hallucinations. It is the content of the experience rather than the experience itself that suggests the possibility of spiritual engagement via open doors. For example, these trips very frequently include emotional and profound interactions with spiritual entities that proselytize New Age spiritualism while specifically denouncing Judeo-Christian beliefs. There is simply no rational explanation for this recurrent phenomenon other than it actually being engagement with spiritual enemies of God. The idea that thousands of people using these substances have experienced the exact same hallucination is not plausible from a biological, psychological, or medical perspective. Providing further evidence of the possibility is the fact that PCP was once commonly referred to as "angel dust" due to users' frequent encounters with spiritual entities who called themselves angels. In my opinion, the beings who were encountered were likely evil, fallen angels masquerading as angels of light.

Dabbling in the Occult

The dangerous behavior of dabbling in the occult frequently opens the door for demonic influence. *Occult* means "hidden," and the fact that there is real power, although demonic in nature, behind occult practices makes it tempting for people to search there for spiritual enlightenment. Because of this risk, God expressly forbids these practices in order to protect his human family from demonic influence. Scripture recounts this:

> *Let no one be found among you who . . . practices divination or sorcery, interprets omens, engages in witchcraft, or casts spells, or who is a medium or spiritist or who consults the dead. Anyone who does these things is detestable to the Lord.*[17]

The occult has become widely accepted in our culture, which is an alarming barometer of where we, collectively, are spiritually. Media depicting ghosts, demons, witches, vampires, and wizards are incredibly popular and big moneymakers. Likewise, Ouija boards, tarot cards, horoscopes, fortune tellers, and séances with spiritual mediums are no longer seen as fringe practices but are widely accepted. Although these practices are pitched as fun and games, God's Spirit warns believers that, in these latter times, the "seducing spirits" behind such practices will cause some to even "depart from the faith" by enticing them to seek knowledge and power from these forbidden sources.[18]

I can't help but wonder if our culture's fascination with the occult may have opened doors to hidden spiritual dimensions, leading to the increase in paranormal phenomena such as UFOs, alien abductions, ghosts, and monsters like Bigfoot, yeti, Loch Ness, Mothman, and chupacabra. For example, some have suggested that the father of modern rocketry, Jack Parsons, and the founder of Scientology, L. Ron Hubbard, may have opened a spiritual door in 1946 when they spent three days in the Mojave Desert performing occult sex magic rituals in an attempt to summon the Thelemic goddess Babalon, so they could birth the Antichrist. Could it be that the alleged UFO crash that occurred in Roswell, New Mexico, the following year, the massive increase in UFO sightings since 1947, and the rise in reported paranormal activity in general are not mere temporal coincidences?

Sexual Sin

The final common means of open-door access to peoples' minds is by sexual sin. Sex is a wonderful gift to humankind from God, which serves to strengthen the bond between married couples and enable procreation to carry out his decree to "be fruitful and multiply." However, sexual perversion—that is, the wrong version—is a very grave sin in the eyes of God. The "sexual revolution" of the 1960s was hailed as a liberation from traditional morals, which taught that sexuality should be exclusively reproductive in nature and confined within the institution of marriage between one man and one woman. This so-called sexual liberation movement led to increased rates of premarital sex, STDs, homosexuality, divorce, and teen pregnancy. Other cultural shifts that resulted include the normalization of pornography, the legalization of abortion, and, in some areas, prostitution, and a general acceptance of sex outside of traditional heterosexual monogamous relationships. Sin is always sold as "liberation" and "freedom" by the Devil, but his version is a *freedom from* God and his perceived restrictive rules rather than a *freedom to* accept responsibility to God and other human imagers of his.

One of the reasons sexual sin is especially abhorrent to God is likely because it is not a victimless crime. By definition, it is a transgression that brings one or more other people into the rebellious activity.

Trauma and sinful practices like those just mentioned essentially grant evil spirits the legal right to enter through the opened doors and have access and more direct influence in peoples' lives. The foothold patients unwittingly grant Satan can soon become a mental stronghold, an impregnable fortress in their mind controlled by enemy forces that becomes first their prison and eventually their tomb.

I urge anyone who has opened such doors to the other side to close them immediately. We will discuss specifics of how to do so in the coming pages. While dramatic spiritual manifestations are rare and demonic possession even rarer, opening such doors does make them more likely. Since you can't put the genie back in the bottle, so to speak, it is most prudent to heed God's warning and be vigilant to guard the doors to the mind by not opening them in the first place.

Strongholds and Towers

The unbelieving slaves of the kingdom of darkness have a dead, nonfunctional spirit and therefore lack spiritual senses and power from God's Spirit to protect their minds from evil spiritual invaders. While these slaves certainly need deliverance from demons, believers transferred to the Kingdom of Light also need deliverance from the strongholds that demons built during the believers' enslavement. Demons may be cast out suddenly, but strongholds are cast down in the same manner they were built—slowly and gradually.

Since demons are disembodied spirits, they constantly search for a house to dwell in. Engaging in sinful habits is like sending out an invitation to them. Demons let in through open doors, metaphorically build a "house" within the mind, known as a stronghold, which becomes ingrained mindsets and behaviors in the minds of those afflicted. Once inside, demons don't just cause temporary chaos; they aim to deeply influence peoples' thinking and actions, leading to their confusion over which thoughts or behaviors belong to them and which come from the demonic influence. Psychotherapy and self-help methods have been developed with the goal of helping people break patterns of negative thinking and behaviors. But without God's supernatural help in this area, patients will only experience temporary moments of thought and behavior modification.

The spiritual battleground of the mind calls for people to utilize spiritual weapons. Those who attempt to fight a spiritual war with only physical or psychological weapons and their own efforts will always fall short of true freedom.

Armed with this knowledge of the battlefield in which their spiritual warfare takes place, people can now develop and implement a detailed counterplan against their demonic foes.

The Counterplan: Offense, Renewal, Defense
Evicting the Enemy, Tearing Down Strongholds, and Replacing Lies

Once slaves born into the kingdom of darkness believe in and receive the gracious offer of salvation from their higher power, they must appropriate their newly delegated authority and power in order to evict their spiritual foes. But when the malevolent spiritual foes are evicted from their mental fortresses, the demonic strongholds of lies remain and act as land mines on the battlefield of the mind. For this reason, the spiritually reborn must go on the offensive to systematically identify the patterns of thought that the enemies have built in their minds over time and then tear down these strongholds. This is a gradual process that requires intentionality and effort. The difference is that once people have transferred their loyalty to the Kingdom of Light, they are then equipped to demolish these remaining strongholds. As Scripture says, "The weapons of our warfare are . . . mighty in God for pulling down strongholds."[19]

People who are freed slaves must cultivate a righteous anger and a strong conviction to annihilate all vacated strongholds of their enemies by assaulting them with the truth of Scripture and the power of the indwelling Spirit of God. Then, those who've been freed must begin to replace false ideas and lies with right thinking, a task made easier by the fact that God created them to be capable of thinking only one thought at a time and thus fortunately unable to hold both right and wrong thoughts concurrently. To do this requires intentionally investing time and effort in thinking about good things. As it is written in the Bible:

> *Fix your thoughts on what is true, and honorable, and right, and pure, and lovely, and admirable. Think about things that are excellent and worthy of praise.*[20]

In response to experiences, thoughts, and behaviors, the human brain has the ability to reorganize and form new neural connections throughout life, a process called *neuroplasticity*. This means that when patients actively shift the way they think, their brain rewires itself, creating new pathways that can lead to lasting changes in behavior and perspective. The verse above is essentially a spiritual admonition that aligns with this scientific principle: What people consistently focus their minds on will shape the structure and function of their brain over time.

When people focus their thoughts on positive, uplifting, and virtuous things, they are actively reshaping the neural pathways in their brains. Repeatedly dwelling on these types of thoughts reinforces these pathways by strengthening the connections between those neurons, making it easier for their minds to return to similar patterns in the future. This is the essence of neuroplasticity—by intentionally choosing to focus on what is good and praiseworthy, as the verse suggests, people can gradually "rewire" their brains to reflect positive, more godly patterns of thinking.

Mind Renewal: An Ongoing Renovation

Next in the demolition job comes the work described in Scripture as "casting down imaginations, and every high thing that exalteth itself against the knowledge of God."[21] The word for "imaginations" in the original Greek, *logismos*, refers to logic or human reasoning. Two types of strongholds founded on lies must be recognized and challenged. Logical strongholds are made up of thoughts that may seem reasonable but limit God's supernatural work. Illogical strongholds, on the other hand, stem from baseless fears or unrealistic worries. The methods of demolishing both strongholds will be addressed later when we discuss the steps of Ruachiatry.

Following this assault against strongholds, the next task is to renew the mind, as the following verse encourages.

> *Don't copy the behavior and customs of this world, but let God transform you into a new person by changing the way you think. Then you will learn to know God's will for you, which is good and pleasing and perfect.*[22]

God, once again, employs neuroplasticity to enable people to forge new pathways in the brain that align with his will. This renewing process not only reflects spiritual growth but also a tangible change in the structure and function of the brain, demonstrating the interplay between faith and the scientific concept of neuroplasticity in personal transformation. The transformation comes from people aligning their thoughts with God's will rather than conforming to the patterns of the world. When people surrender their will and allow God to change the way they think—focusing on spiritual truths and rejecting worldly behaviors—this reshaping of their thought patterns triggers the gradual, but often dramatic, personal transformation. Scientifically, this aligns with how neuroplasticity enables people to break free from old, negative thought patterns and adopt new, healthier ways of thinking. These words of encouragement from Scripture apply:

Since you have heard about Jesus and have learned the truth that comes from him, throw off your old sinful nature and your former way of life, which is corrupted by lust and deception. Instead, let the Spirit renew your thoughts and attitudes.[23]

The Greek word for "renew," *ananeoo*, means to be remade by an inward renovation that implies an ongoing process. When God gets ready to change people, he first changes how they think. Many people today erroneously believe their circumstances must change before their minds can change, but the fact of the matter is just the opposite. Psychiatrist Viktor Frankl introduced the concept of attitudinal values, proposing that despite adverse circumstances and suffering not of their choosing, people still possess the ability to choose their attitude toward their situation. This radical acceptance of "whatever is, is best, because it is the will of God" will be discussed in greater detail in Chapter 13, which outlines the first three steps of Ruachiatry.[24]

Many faiths offer a vital path to renewal. In Islam, *tazkiyah* focuses on purifying the thoughts. In Judaism, *tikkun middot* refers to transforming the mind and heart through a refinement of character. Additionally, Hinduism's yoga and Buddhism's *vipassana* transform through insight.

In Christianity, it is God's Spirit who initiates and enables the renewal of peoples' minds with a two-pronged approach. First, the Holy Spirit must work from the outside in, exposing peoples' minds to Christ-centered truth through the gospel, Bible study, and spiritual meditation. Second, the Spirit must work from the inside out by breaking peoples' formerly hard hearts bent on self-will exalted above God's will and by fostering humility. People are admonished by Scripture not to follow the desires they had when they were ignorant of God, an ignorance that was actually a willful rejection of God's truth that formerly enslaved them to harmful passions.[25] The renewal of the mind is essential for the transformation that can free people from these destructive desires.

Building New Watchtowers and Guarding the Gates

After tearing down strongholds and experiencing a renewal of their mind, people must get down to the work of protecting the battlefield of their mind by building new watchtowers with the words of God as the new foundation and wisdom bestowed by God as the walls. These new replacement strongholds grow more formidable with every brick of wisdom obtained from the study of holy Scripture.

The next task in shoring up the defenses of the mind is keeping watch, being especially vigilant not to unwittingly open any gates by means of willful disobedience to God. Only with the peace of God that comes with his pardon and reconciliation can freed slaves adequately guard their minds and hearts.[26]

In Christianity, believers must regularly use the mind of Christ, which is continually renewed in them by the Holy Spirit. The holy Scriptures now give them truth to better recognize demonic deception, and their reborn spirit submitted to God grants them discernment. But it's important to remember that Satan does not abandon the battlefield. Instead, he continues his assault with more stealthy tactics. Going forward, believers must realize that not all of the thoughts that enter their mind are their own and that Satan wants them to think his voice is their voice. There are four possible sources of the thoughts that people might experience—self, secular, demonic, or God's Spirit.

The minds of believers are like walled cities that demons are not allowed to enter. In his novel *The Holy War*, John Bunyan describes five gates in the walled city of Mansoul, each corresponding to a specific faculty of a person—the eye gate, the ear gate, the mouth gate, the nose gate, and the feel gate—which Bunyan describes must all be carefully guarded so that Diabolus (the Devil) cannot enter and control Mansoul by deception, temptation, and sin.[27] I often advise patients to consider that just as they would not dream of eating trash, they should likewise not watch trash, listen to trash, speak trash, smell trash, or play with trash in order to chase a certain feeling.

But even if the gates to the believers' minds are relatively well guarded, demons can still essentially bypass this protection by lobbing deceptive thought bombs over the wall. If people then entertain the thoughts, the bomb metaphorically explodes, creating an opening in the wall to their minds, giving demons the legal right to enter and start rebuilding a stronghold. One way people can know if a particular thought may be from the enemy is if it is intrusive and what psychiatrists call *egodystonic* (in conflict with their true self and God's indwelling Spirit).

Satan is a thief who stealthily becomes an unwelcome intruder in peoples' minds, producing thoughts lacking the fruits of God's Spirit and characterized by pride, condemnation, accusation, dissension, and discord toward other humans. Also, in my experience, all-or-nothing, black-or-white, and always-and-never thinking patterns may be sown by spiritual interlopers to ensnare and discourage patients. Fortunately, patients should be able to distinguish thoughts from God's Spirit from those sent by their spiritual enemies by weighing them against the godly traits of love, joy, peace, patience, kindness, goodness, faithfulness, gentleness, and self-control.[28]

As discussed earlier in this chapter, the human conscience is not infallible. It can be influenced and shaped by various factors, such as upbringing, culture, and personal beliefs. But the conscience serves an important function in the spiritual life of people by acting as a window between the soul and spirit that can be a powerful tool for guiding their moral and ethical decisions when enlightened by holy Scripture and empowered by God's Spirit.

Satanic Condemnation vs. Holy Conviction

The conscience must be regularly calibrated by the guiding light of holy Scripture and God's Spirit. A voice of conviction when people miss the mark is always from the Holy Spirit's influence on their conscience, intending to drive them back to God in repentance. People can discern the voice of God's Spirit by the fact that it will never contradict his holy Scripture.

A voice of condemnation, on the other hand, could be either from the Accuser or the false self that he has cultivated in a person over time by means of lies. In either case, the Accuser's intention is to drive believers away from God, producing shame and despair. Having been freed from the death penalty of sin by the sacrifice of God's Messiah on the cross, believers should confidently remind themselves that, as Scripture says, "now there is no condemnation for those who belong to Christ Jesus."[29]

In addition to shame and despair through condemnation, another tactic the Accuser employs is trying to convince people that their issues are their identity, especially regarding mental illness. For example, I have never heard any patient utter in clinical practice, "I am hypertension" or "I am diabetes." But many times, I hear patients say, "I *am* depressed" or "I *am* anxious" rather than saying, "I am John or Jane Doe who currently suffers from major depressive disorder or generalized anxiety disorder." It is not psychologically healthy for patients to identify as their illness; rather, they need to accept their illness as an unfortunate state of affliction, or even as an enemy separate from their being.

Secular thoughts are the voice of the flesh, responding to the enticements of the world system through music, movies, sports, gaming, and mind-altering substances that entertain or distract patients. But, as Scripture tells us, "The world offers only a craving for physical pleasure, a craving for everything we see, and pride in our achievements and possessions."[30]

Awakening Spiritual Senses

When slaves are freed by a spiritual rebirth, they undergo a profound spiritual transformation that changes their perception of the world, themselves, and God. This transformation is like acquiring new spiritual senses that go beyond the five physical senses of sight, hearing, touch, taste, and smell. These new spiritual senses allow believers to see with faith, hear God's voice, feel his presence, taste his goodness, sense the fragrance of Christ, and have new desires in line with God's will.

But this new set of senses needs to be sharpened by practice. For instance, people must practice seeing beyond the physical realm, recognizing spiritual truths and the reality of the unseen world. They must likewise develop an increasing sensitivity to the voice of God, whether through scripture, prayer, or the guidance of the Holy Spirit. In developing their spiritual hearing, the faithful must practice identifying and then silencing thoughts from the secular, the demonic, and the false self so that they can clearly hear the Holy Spirit. Additionally, those who are spiritually reborn gain spiritual discernment to sense the difference between truth and error, good and evil. Their spiritual appetite also changes, as they find themselves with a new hunger and thirst for righteousness as worldly desires begin to fade. These changes are a testament to the powerful work of God's Spirit, leading believers into a deeper and more vibrant relationship with their higher power. People should remind themselves of who they now are with the indwelling Holy Spirit, who testifies with their spirit that they are indeed children of God.[31]

Discerning the Spirits

Satan's plan for the battlefield of the mind hasn't changed much over thousands of years:

The Devil sends the spirit of fear, leading to an anxious mind, whereas God sends his Spirit of power and love, leading to a sound mind.[32]

The Devil sends a spirit of perversion and sensuality, leading to a debased and carnal mind, whereas God sends his renewing Holy Spirit, leading to a spiritual mind focused on the things of God.[33]

The Devil sends the spirit of the world to intoxicate and enflame lustful passions, whereas God sends his Spirit of hope, leading to a sober, self-controlled mind.[34]

The Devil sends the spirit of delusion, leading to a psychotic mind, whereas God sends his Spirit of healing, leading to restoration of a right mind.[35]

Victory on the battlefield of the mind can be achieved by people tearing down mental strongholds, renewing their minds, building new watchtowers based on the wisdom of the words of God, and then vigorously guarding their thought life, as the mind and heart control their actions and, ultimately, their destiny. The key to maintaining pure thoughts is for believers to immerse themselves in holy Scripture, which is alive and has the power to cleanse and guide.[36] A God-controlled mind will influence speech, sight, and actions, aligning one's life with God's will.

In this ongoing spiritual war, people must be aware that their brain processes, their mind interprets, but their spirit gives purpose. When all three are aligned, human beings are not only whole but free—free to live the life for which they were created, free to fulfill their destiny as imagers of God.

SPIRITUAL SOLUTIONS

12

RUACHIATRY: THE PROFOUND SPIRITUAL COMPONENT OF MEDICINE

We are not human beings having a spiritual experience.
We are spiritual beings having a human experience.

—PIERRE TEILHARD DE CHARDIN, FRENCH
PHILOSOPHER AND JESUIT PRIEST

The Limits of Modern Medicine

The field of medicine has made unprecedented scientific advances in the diagnosis and treatment of illness in the twentieth and twenty-first centuries thus far. Yet, despite these advances, both the prevalence and severity of many medical conditions, especially psychiatric disorders, appear to be increasing. For example, a study in the *Journal of Abnormal Psychology* found that among young people aged twelve to twenty-five years old, the rates of severe psychological distress, major depressive episodes, and suicidal ideation, attempts, and deaths increased between the mid-2000s and 2017.[1]

The issue of the increased prevalence of mental disorders in young people is especially alarming given the fact that it has been known for decades that presentation of psychiatric illness at a younger age increases the likelihood that the disorder will be both chronic and severe in nature. I share the opinion of many others that societal factors, such as electronics and social media, are playing a large role in this presentation.

For those who are older, the outlook hasn't necessarily improved either. The National Institutes of Health reports that in the past twenty years there has been an increase among patients over fifty in the prevalence of three medical illnesses—cancer, diabetes, and stroke.[2] It is likely that better available treatments in recent years have allowed patients to live longer with chronic disease, but this has, in turn, led to increasing states of disability as patients age. In other words, today a longer lifespan does not necessarily equate to an improved quality of life and functionality; it often leads to the exact opposite.

While there is ongoing debate regarding the reasons for this increasing prevalence and severity observed in many medical and psychiatric conditions, I believe that part of the explanation lies in a notable shift in focus from evaluating and treating the whole person to focusing primarily on the biological, somatic components of illness. The biological approach dominated general medicine for much of the twentieth century until George Engel, a pioneer in psychosomatic medicine, proposed the biopsychosocial model in 1977, in which he suggested that "all three levels, biological, psychological, and social, must be taken into account in every healthcare task."[3] This more holistic approach was standard for several decades before waning. But it took a back seat once again around the turn of the century as the proliferation of technology, scientific discoveries, and knowledge set in.

I first witnessed the strong shift to the biological emphasis in medical practice when I was deciding between various psychiatric residency training programs in the mid-1990s, during a period often called "the decade of the brain" in medical circles. Some programs touted that they emphasized burgeoning biological psychiatry in their training, while others emphasized traditional psychodynamic principles, and still others proffered a hybrid approach. It is now clear that biological psychiatry has won the day in the twenty-first century, overtaking the psychoanalytic approach, popularized by Freud, that dominated psychiatry for much of the twentieth century. Freud himself assented to a truth that was taken for granted back then and seemingly is not even recognized by many today—that humans are spiritual beings. In fact, Freud once asserted: "Humanity has always known it possesses a spirit; it was my task to show it has instincts as well."[4] Perhaps it is time we remember this forgotten truth— that a spiritual component to human existence was once accepted as self-evident by almost all cultures throughout history.

The Forgotten Spiritual Dimension

The main problem with the field of medicine's shift of focus to the biological realm in general is its insufficiency. It has left patients with three out of the four components of a proposed biopsychosocial-spiritual model of disease either under-addressed or altogether neglected. In a biological paradigm, the only thing that makes the medical doctor different from a veterinarian is the clientele.

Adding the spiritual component to Engel's proposed biopsycho-social model has been suggested since at least the 1990s but has never gained widespread acceptance nor incorporation into standard medical education or practice.[5] This is puzzling, since there are now more than 3,000 quantitative scientific studies on religion, spirituality, and health, the majority of which suggest that religion and spirituality lead to better outcomes regarding physical, psychological, and social health.[6] Dr. Harold Koenig, a psychiatrist colleague of mine at Duke University, is a leading researcher in this area of religion, spirituality, and health, and he suggests that the reason religion is still an important part of the lives of many well-educated and informed modern people today is that it may serve the purpose of preserving health.[7]

Barriers to Spiritual Integration in Medicine

So why, then, hasn't the spiritual component of patients' lives been widely incorporated into medical assessments and treatment? I believe the reasons for this are complex but largely due to a few primary factors.

First, physicians are reluctant to discuss these spiritual issues with patients because medical training dictates that doctors allow patients to make autonomous decisions regarding their healthcare. So, physicians have understandable concerns about interjecting any undue influence or coercion into the relationship.

Second, there is a general lack of clarity and understanding surrounding the terms *religion* and *spirituality*. This leads to a common posture of indifference regarding any treatment that crosses into these realms.

Third, most physicians are admittedly ill-equipped to employ religion and spirituality assessment or treatments due to lack of formal education and training in their medical curricula. A systematic literature review of sixty-one papers regarding doctors discussing religion and spirituality with their patients found that most physicians: 1) infrequently engage in these discussions with patients unless patients have a terminal illness and 2) prefer referral to a chaplain rather than engaging personally with their patients on these matters.[8]

In addition to the inconsistent nature of physicians' interactions with their patients regarding religion and spirituality issues, the literature review also found that many twenty-first century practitioners are both ill-equipped by their education and training and lack the requisite time needed to evaluate and address spiritual concerns of patients.[9] For example, we've probably all experienced the reality that primary care physicians in the outpatient office setting often experience time constraints. While conscientious primary care providers may refer their patients to mental health practitioners, evidence indicates that most patients often do not follow up regarding the referral.[10] The dirty little secret is that even though mental health referrals are made by primary care providers in good faith, there is, in actuality, a fundamental problem with access to care due to a paucity of qualified mental health practitioners in most nonurban communities. Access to needed mental healthcare services is further restricted by the fact that many mental health practitioners have elected not to participate in health insurance reimbursement plans due to the onerous management of their patients' care associated with the plans and the lower reimbursement that participants receive for services.

The Consequences of a Sick Care System

These limitations to accessing timely, expert, and affordable mental healthcare predictably result in psychological issues being undertreated or neglected. As a result, the trend I've noticed over the past twenty-eight years is that by the time patients reach my psychiatric practice, the symptoms they initially describe have become increasingly severe.

The same phenomenon has long been observed in somatic illnesses. For example, when patients with physical maladies lack access to care for whatever reason, they also tend to present with very severe and advanced cases of illness when they finally do see a healthcare provider, often in emergency departments of large urban teaching hospitals. I have also witnessed this firsthand while providing healthcare in Third World nations.

While *preventive medicine* and *holistic healthcare* have been buzz-words since at least the 1990s, their implementation into standard practice has not occurred, because the system that is in place simply does not reward best practice. *Health* is increasingly defined as merely the absence or management of disease symptoms. This stands in stark contrast to the World Health Organization's definition: "Health is a state of complete physical, mental and social well-being."[11] The current healthcare system in the United States could be more aptly described as a "sick care system," in which doctors attempt to improve their patients' symptoms rather than treat underlying causes, one of which is the routinely neglected spiritual component.

In the past, healthcare practitioners had the luxury of spending more time with patients. They were often able to learn more about a patient's psychological makeup, social supports, and spirituality. But the landscape in medical practice has changed drastically for most providers over the past thirty years, leading to shorter office visits and increased patient volume. The reasons for this shift are also complex and multifaceted, but obvious sources are 1) the effects of the proliferation of managed care in the reimbursement and delivery of healthcare services, 2) the increased prevalence of medical and psychiatric illnesses, 3) the rising elder population, who have more chronic illnesses needing regular management, and 4) patients' increased willingness to seek healthcare due to the availability of scientifically advanced treatments that are generally more efficacious and better tolerated.

We in the field of medicine have forgotten our historical roots. For millennia, those bearing the mantle of healer in virtually all societies and cultures—be they called shaman, priest, medicine man, or witch doctor—have employed spiritual practices along with medicinal ones to heal their patients. With today's focus on scientific and technological advancements, spiritual problems are rarely addressed in the physician's office. But, as evidence clearly shows, this is not because patients lack interest in having them addressed. More likely, it is because physicians are not equipped through their medical education and residency training to adequately address these issues. Outside of the inpatient hospital setting, physicians rarely refer patients to chaplains or pastoral counselors. Instead, solutions for the spiritual component of a malady are usually sought by the patient via self-referral to alternative and complementary medicine practitioners, most of whom do not share the same faith traditions and practices as their patients.

What exactly is this spiritual component of existence with which we physicians seem to have lost touch? Simply put, the spirit is that divine, nonphysical, eternal foundation of being that allows us to commune with the transcendent and search for meaning, especially in the context of suffering as in illness and death. However, if twenty-first-century medical practice tends to emphasize the physical and neglect the soul, then I think it is fair to postulate that the spirit is forgotten altogether. This is largely because medical practitioners are trained scientists taught that spiritual matters belong in the realm of religion and theology, not science. The overlooked reality is that the spiritual component of human existence is foundational to our being, a core element upon which the body, mind, will, and emotions rest. If the spirit is sick, it only stands to reason that it is a matter of time before the body and soul are negatively affected as well. Likewise, even if the body and/or soul are sick, having a healthy spiritual foundation will prove essential in coping with disease and aiding in recovery.

An aging population with increasing life expectancy will struggle with progressive chronic illnesses. Chronic illness is a burden that patients will likely have increasingly less capacity to bear as they age, leading to more suffering and diminishing quality of life. Shouldn't physicians employ all possible avenues of treatment when helping people find meaning in their suffering and in their struggles to thrive? While overhauling the existing healthcare system is not tenable, the initiation of incremental, intentional changes is not only realistic in its scope but also necessary as concerned physicians battle for the soul of medicine.

Ruachiatry: Healing Through the Spirit

Having presented evidence supporting the reality of a spiritual world in which an invisible war is being waged, it is my opinion that physicians and other healthcare providers should be taught and trained to incorporate spiritual realities into their practices. Occasional referral to chaplains or pastoral counselors is an insufficient strategy for this fight; it's like showing up to a gunfight with a knife.

For millennia, humankind has proven to be innately religious. Furthermore, there are universal spiritual principles common to most major religions, which makes the incorporation of a spiritual assessment and intervention into the medical field a reasonable proposal. This addition of the spiritual component to the treatment of body and soul is what I call *Ruachiatry*, a term derived from a combination of the Hebrew word *ruach*, meaning "spirit," and the Greek *iatreia*, meaning "healing."

The real question is, how can physicians practically address the spiritual components of physical or mental illness in the clinical setting? It begins with fully comprehending that they are on foreign turf and that the battle for healing and health is not against flesh and blood.

Physicians and healthcare workers are accustomed to primarily fighting diseases and disorders with biological weapons, such as medications, surgeries, and physical therapies. Mental health practitioners employ psychological therapies as well. But since the battle with the spiritual is not against flesh and blood, the weaponry needed is understandably neither physical nor psychological in nature.[12] The battle to help patients requires spiritual weapons with which most healers are unfamiliar. In fact, the only specialty in the broad field of medicine that both acknowledges a spiritual component to the manifestation of illnesses and employs a spiritual treatment is the field of addiction medicine. So, drawing upon some of its foundational principles seems a logical starting point.

Alcoholics Anonymous, the basic textbook of the eponymous program that was first published in 1939 and is also known as "the Big Book," states that alcoholics suffer from a spiritual disease:

> *For we have been not only mentally and physically ill, we have been spiritually sick. When the spiritual malady is overcome, we straighten out mentally and physically.*[13]

For more than eighty years, the Alcoholics Anonymous (A.A.) program and its Twelve Steps have proven to be a very effective intervention for alcohol use disorder, a malady that previously had a very grim prognosis. According to an analysis of twenty-seven studies conducted on 10,565 participants by researchers from the Stanford University School of Medicine in 2020, A.A. was nearly always found to be more effective in achieving abstinence from alcohol than established treatments, such as cognitive behavioral psychotherapy. Furthermore, most studies showed that A.A. participation lowered healthcare costs, leading the authors to conclude that the program "probably produces substantial healthcare cost savings among people with alcohol use disorder."[14] The implications of this study are huge, especially if similar principles could be applied to other physical and mental illnesses.

Here is where the comparable 12 Steps of Ruachiatry come into play. In my outpatient suburban private practice, my team has studied the effects of applying these twelve steps to patients suffering from major depression that is unresponsive to three or more past antidepressant medication treatments, which are considered the standard of care in psychiatry. Patients in our clinic who met these criteria and who consented to participate were told they would be involved in an ongoing study to evaluate the effectiveness of a new, nonmedical treatment incorporating spirituality.

During the course of the twelve-week Ruachiatry trial, no changes were made in the participants' medication or psychotherapy regimens. Participants agreed to utilize the proposed spiritual treatment of the 12 Steps of Ruachiatry on a daily basis and to have a weekly session with the Ruachiatry coach, a psychiatric nurse practitioner trained in this model, to facilitate their step work and assess their progress. The results so far in our ongoing trial have been overwhelmingly positive. For example, in our initial cohort, the average score on the Beck Depression Inventory, Second Edition (BDI-II), at the beginning of the study was 31.5, considered to be in the severe range of symptoms. At the conclusion of twelve weeks, the average BDI-II score had dropped from 31.5 to 16.2—a 47.6 percent decrease—considered to be in the mild range of symptoms. These initial findings highlight the need for larger, multisite, controlled trials. We will gladly make our protocols available to any clinician upon request for professional use.

Incorporation of these steps into clinical practice could become a reality if the biopsychosocial-spiritual approach gains wider acceptance and if medical schools and residency programs are intentional about incorporating this approach in their education and training. Because many of the steps of Ruachiatry can be intimidating, in a clinical setting it is advisable to consider having Ruachiatry-trained coaches help patients work through them. To get traction, patients will need to schedule regular consultations, preferably at least once weekly, initially. Most physicians and advanced practice clinicians lack the time and space in their busy schedules to accommodate these requirements. However, if they are willing and available, these clinicians would be preferable due to their position of authority in the medical hierarchy and the likelihood that they already have a trusted relationship with their patients. But other members of the healthcare team, including nurses, therapists, or even potentially medical assistants, could become trained and certified Ruachiatry coaches. The American Ruachiatry Association will soon offer a standardized curriculum for interested medical professionals to become a certified Ruachiatry coach to better serve their patients' unaddressed spiritual needs in a clinical setting.

Clinicians may refer their patients to the website *www. Ruachiatry.org* for resources about the 12 Steps of Ruachiatry. There, those interested in joining or starting an in-person or Zoom support group can learn about Paracletus Groups, which exist to support individuals in their journey toward health recovery through the 12-step process and the principles of Ruachiatry. Guided by the concept of Paracletus, an advocate called to comfort and strengthen, groups provide a compassionate, inclusive community where members of all faiths can find hope, healing, and connection. By integrating holistic healthcare with spiritual growth, groups empower individuals to better navigate health challenges, embrace a higher power of their understanding, and practice preventive wellness. The mission is to walk alongside each member as a supportive ally, fostering clarity, resilience, and a renewed sense of purpose.

In Chapters 13 through 15, I briefly describe each of the 12 Steps of Ruachiatry. In summarizing the action of each step, I use the past tense and "we," an intentional detail modeled after the language of the well-documented Twelve Steps from Alcoholics Anonymous.[15] My hope in presenting these descriptions is to provide a reference tool that will help patients who are on their own spiritual journey find healing. It is also my hope that these chapters inspire health-care providers to explore this uncharted territory with open minds and to answer the call to offer patients a more complete path to healing by embracing the spiritual dimension of health.

Finally, while Ruachiatry is rooted in a Judeo-Christian under-standing of spiritual healing, it acknowledges that spiritual healing is a global pursuit expressed through many traditions and prac-tices, and it strives to honor the diversity of human beliefs while focusing on a shared goal: wholeness. By exploring these diverse approaches, we see a common thread: Healing is most effective when it addresses the deeper layers of human existence, not just the surface symptoms. As a psychiatrist, I respect the autonomy of each individual to choose their path. Ruachiatry is not about imposing any set of spiritual beliefs but empowering patients to explore their own spirituality.

Many faiths and cultures also recognize the importance of treating the whole person—body, soul, and spirit. For example, Ayurvedic medicine, one of the world's oldest holistic healing sys-tems, focuses on balancing the mind, body, and spirit through diet, herbal remedies, detoxification, and meditation. Furthermore, Buddhism offers meditation as a path to transcend suffering, while Islam emphasizes that the condition of the heart affects the entire being, with spiritual purification (*tazkiyah*) being as crucial to health as any physical treatment.

Ruachiatry provides a new holistic framework where patients can draw from their faith traditions—or discover new ones—to address the spiritual contributors to their illness. Widespread adoption of the principles of Ruachiatry could finally move medicine toward a true biopsychosocial-spiritual model that could benefit all those suffering from illness.

13

STEPS 1–3: ACCEPTANCE, SEARCHING, AND SUBMISSION

The journey toward healing, as outlined in the principles of Ruachiatry, begins with a series of three foundational steps—acceptance, searching, and submission—that lay the groundwork for addressing the spiritual dimensions of illness and prepare the patient for transformation.

Step 1: Acceptance and Commitment

We accepted that we were powerless over our illness and made a decision to take a stand.

Embracing the Reality of Illness

The first part of Step 1 concerns accepting the reality of a state of suffering due to physical or mental maladies, including their potential spiritual components. This sounds easy on the surface, but in actual practice, it is very difficult for two reasons. First, patients are born spiritually blind and then face opposition to experiencing a spiritual awakening. Secondly, often there is a process of grieving the loss of health and functionality that patients must work through. There is a reason that acceptance is the final stage of grief, following denial, anger, bargaining, and depression; it often takes some time to reach.[1]

Many religious faiths share this concept of acceptance. In Islam, acceptance is reflected in *tawakkul* (trust in Allah), encouraging believers to accept their trials as part of divine wisdom. Buddhism teaches *samma ditthi* (right view), accepting the truth of suffering (*dukkha*) as the first Noble Truth, while Hinduism emphasizes *santosha* (contentment), accepting one's current state as a basis for spiritual growth. In Christianity, believers must first accept they are sinners both by birth and choice and then acknowledge their need for divine intervention.

Acknowledging Powerlessness

If patients had any significant power over their illness, they likely would not be seeking the help of a physician in the first place. Verbalizing their powerlessness helps drive home the reality that the problem with which patients grapple is severe in nature, necessitating outside expert help. As a result, when patients present themselves to healthcare practitioners, the clinician's initial task is to meet them where they are in the process and then plan to move them toward acceptance of their illness and suffering as quickly as possible.

Even though patients may be powerless in the face of their suffering, they do retain the power to choose their attitude about it. It is in their enduring of suffering that patients actualize what psychiatrist Viktor Frankl called "attitudinal values," which bring meaning to patients' lives, he said, when they are "confronted by a destiny toward which they can act only by acceptance." As long as patients remain alive, Frankl posited, they are responsible for realizing values, "even if these be only attitudinal values."[2]

Human life has a task quality to it, and it becomes more meaningful as tasks become more difficult. This means suffering lends itself to great opportunities for spiritual and psychological growth. King Solomon, the leader of ancient Israel renowned for his wisdom, discovered that many of life's pursuits were a vain waste of time, but he did find that one thing is good: "For people . . . to accept their lot in life . . . ," he said, "this is indeed a gift from God."[3] The physician must help patients accept that their unique and very personal tasks constitute a mission of sorts that is affirmed by a calling. Patients not only have a responsibility for fulfilling their life tasks but also a responsibility to a taskmaster.

Drawing Strength from Faith

Saul of Tarsus was a first-century Jewish rabbi who was an ardent persecutor of early Jewish followers of Jesus until he was blinded on the road to Damascus and encountered the risen Jesus. The arrogant and brash Pharisee, named after the first King of Israel, then himself became a follower of Jesus, who changed Saul's name to Paul, meaning "small, humble." Paul went on to author the majority of the New Testament and travel throughout the Roman Empire on missionary journeys spreading the good news of Jesus's resurrection, winning converts, and founding churches along the way. Paul believed that the spiritual component of peoples' suffering must be fought with spiritual weapons, and he gave the most systematic approach in his letter to the church at Ephesus around 61 AD.

In conclusion, be strong in the Lord [draw your strength from Him and be empowered through your union with Him] and in the power of His [boundless] might. Put on the full armor of God [for His precepts are like the splendid armor of a heavily armed soldier], so that you may be able to [successfully] stand up against all the schemes and the strategies and the deceits of the Devil. For our struggle is not against flesh and blood [contending only with physical opponents], but against the rulers, against the powers, against the world forces of this [present] darkness, against the spiritual forces of wickedness in the heavenly [supernatural] places. Therefore, put on the complete armor of God, so that you will be able to [successfully] resist and stand your ground in the evil day [of danger], and having done everything [that the crisis demands], to stand firm [in your place, fully prepared, immovable, victorious].[4]

Paul's admonition to "be strong in the Lord and in the power of His might" is at once the remedy for our patients' powerlessness over their illness and organically leads the patient to Step 2, in which they decide, after an earnest search, who this higher power is to them. Clearly, patients with ongoing suffering despite medical treatment need further assistance from some higher power. Paul asserts that the God of the Bible is able and willing to provide his strength to patients in the midst of their medical maladies.

Deciding to Stand Firm

The second part of Step 1 concerns the decision to take a stand, a concept that is also derived from St. Paul's admonition to the believers in Ephesus. Patients must come to terms with the reality that they live on a battleground, not a playground; they are in a lifelong fight, which they did not start, with powerful unseen enemies, who are ruthless and fight dirty. Before patients accept the reality of the fierce foe of disease and the possibility of unseen forces behind it, they are defenseless and unwittingly wounded in this invisible war that rages around them. The first stage of recovery from these wounds is the decision to take a stand and take all that it has to dish out. In a military battle, a stand is a defensive position to hold one's ground when facing a formidable opponent. Needless to say, one cannot fight when he or she is knocked down. So, metaphorically speaking, the medical clinician first helps the patient get up off the mat.

In a boxing match, the fight continues despite knockdowns, as long as each boxer gets up off the mat. Ultimately, the last one standing wins. In the classic film *Rocky II*, after getting knocked down by his world champion opponent, the weary and outmatched challenger, Rocky Balboa, says to his trainer between rounds, "I ain't going down no more."[5] In the first of the 12 Steps of Ruachiatry, patients must embrace a similar posture.

This decision to take a stand is difficult, because, like Rocky, many patients are weary and feel like throwing in the towel. But this is when perseverance and determination are needed most. By displaying genuine peace amid suffering that is unjust and chronic, and demonstrating that they can stand when most around them are falling, patients can then carry the message of hope and encouragement to others.[6]

This is also when a healthcare professional has the wonderful privilege of coming alongside suffering patients, helping to carry their burdens in the midst of their battle and instilling hope in the process. Patients learn that they are not alone in their fight and that they have a skilled, understanding, knowledgeable, and encouraging coach in their corner. Physicians cannot fight the battles *for* their patients, but they can stand alongside them and fight *with* them.

However, as helpful as physicians can be in their patients' fights with illness, physicians are neither omnipotent nor omniscient. So, it makes sense that if someone possessing these traits is available, it would be wise to earnestly seek out that individual. Holy Scripture states that God draws all people to himself, and he will use adversity to help patients realize that they need a higher power to aid them in their fight. Earnestly seeking this higher power who, Scripture says, "helps the fallen and lifts those bent beneath their loads," is the task of Step 2.[7]

Step 2: Searching

We earnestly embarked on a journey to fulfill our personal responsibility to discover the truth regarding a spiritual power greater than ourselves who could give us hope of either restoring our health or enabling us to cope with our sickness.

After making the decision to stand firm, patients are now ready to prepare to reenter the battlefield and successfully stand their ground. Having read the first twelve chapters of this book, you have hopefully come to an acknowledgment of the reality of the spiritual realm and the spiritual unseen war that rages on around us. Having a physician in your corner is a great start, but that alone is wholly inadequate to defeat our powerful spiritual foes.

Recognizing the Need for a Higher Power

Patients need a power higher than that of modern medicine.

An example of this truth is seen in the Hebrew Old Testament when King Asa of Judah developed a severe foot disease. He did not receive a cure, the Scripture says, because "he did not seek the Lord's help but turned only to his physicians."[8] Patients should not only seek appropriate medical help for their maladies but also make a decision to discover who, exactly, this higher spiritual power, whom most people call God, is—and then humbly appeal to him for help. Essentially, patients must become willing to embark on a fearless journey to truth, wherever that may lead. Contrary to what our relativistic, postmodern culture insists, truth is both knowable and demonstrably exclusive, not relative in nature. In other words, 2 + 2 = 5 is not your truth while 2 + 2 = 4 is my truth, because 2 + 2 = 4 is *the* exclusive and objectively verifiable truth, regardless of one's feelings or opinions.

An important point here: Patients are only going to go as far in this spiritual battle as their god is able to help them go. I have heard of patients who, while in substance use disorder recovery, state that their higher power is a house plant or the ocean. As a physician and therapist, I have been trained to be nonjudgmental toward patients; however, statements such as these always make me ponder whether the patient has, in fact, *earnestly embarked on a journey to fulfill their personal responsibility to discover the truth regarding a spiritual power greater than themselves.*

Seeking Truth with Earnestness

The all-important question of whether there is a God is the foundation upon which one's very worldview rests. If patients do not believe in a higher power or do not ascribe to a particular religious faith, they likely cannot even realize that they are in a war that has left them wounded. Or they may realize that they've been wounded but do not understand the spiritual powers behind it. As a result, they are more likely to blame others, themselves, or circumstances for their hurt. Furthermore, they're more likely to seek the wrong remedy. The longer this goes on, the more wounds they accumulate. Therefore, it is wise for patients to earnestly seek the truth, and once they find it, follow it wholeheartedly. Only then can they begin the healing process.

In the course of taking a spiritual history, if physicians find that their patients do not identify a higher power, the physician should strongly suggest that they earnestly embark on a journey to identify their higher power and to accept that this is their responsibility alone. If patients decline to do so, the physician must respect their autonomy in this regard but also should politely inquire as to the reasons they are reluctant to do so.

Here I'll offer a cautionary word about patients who label themselves "spiritual but not religious" (SBNR). While many in our culture embrace this view because it seems more open-minded, tolerant, and independent than some religious views, scientific literature suggests that it does not hold the same health benefits. For example, a 2013 multinational study involving 8,318 medical outpatients found that those who identified themselves as SBNR were more likely to experience a major depressive episode over the next twelve months than those with a secular view.[9] Another study in 2013, comprised of 7,403 people in England, found that those who described themselves as SBNR were more likely to have used or been dependent on drugs and to have generalized anxiety disorder and phobias than those who were neither religious nor spiritual.[10]

My concern for SBNR patients is that, rather than getting the help they believe they are seeking from a benevolent higher power, they may unwittingly be receiving influence from malevolent spirits who are bent on *causing* medical and psychological problems. My personal experience and my clinical experience with thousands of patients over the years have taught me that genuine, open-minded seekers of truth will not be denied. Scripture in both the Old and New Testaments of the Bible promises this as well.[11] But seekers must put forth the effort, and laziness in this regard will likely lead to neither the help they seek nor the protection they need against their formidable demonic foes. The goal is to seek and find the omnipotent Highest Power to help them.

If, on the other hand, patients do identify a higher power, physicians should briefly inquire as to how they came to that conclusion. By doing so, physicians can judge whether patients were earnest in their search or the degree to which their decision might be based on cultural factors or even coercion. Patients cannot win this fight by utilizing a faith they have merely inherited; patients must have a faith of their own, born from a personal experience with the transcendent.

Once one expresses intellectual assent of a power greater than oneself, the logical question is, Which power? It is each individual's responsibility to thoroughly search this matter out and decide for themselves who or what their higher power is. If it is "God," which god is it?

In Judeo-Christian tradition, God has many names, because the nature of his being is so multidimensional. And since his ways are so much higher than our ways, knowing more about his nature through his names can enable patients to draw closer to the divine.[12] One name of God that is particularly relevant to Ruachiatry is Jehovah-Rapha.[13] *Jehovah* means "I am," referring to God's self-existent, eternal nature, and the Hebrew term *rapha* derives from a root meaning "to heal." While I advocate for the autonomy of patients to decide on their higher power, I strongly encourage them to earnestly embark on a journey to discover who exactly this higher power is and to at least examine the claims of the omnipotent "God who heals,"[14] whether struggling with physical, psychological, and/or spiritual maladies.

The Soldier's First Piece of Battle Gear

Once patients have identified a specific higher power, they are ready to begin putting on the spiritual armor that God makes available, demonstrating their commitment to fighting this spiritual battle.

Only soldiers put on armor. The six pieces of this spiritual armor are described in the New Testament book of Ephesians Chapter 6.

The first piece is the metaphorical Belt of Truth. The Apostle Paul was no doubt inspired by the armor of the elite Roman soldiers of his day when he described the armor necessary for spiritual warfare. The soldier's belt was the first piece of armor he would put on, and it was the foundation of his defensive outfit that held his only offensive weapon, the sword. The belt also supported the rest of his armor and allowed the soldier to tuck in his tunic and run when necessary. Similarly, truth is the foundation upon which our spiritual battles rest, making it imperative that patients put forth the effort to find it. Having earnestly sought and then identified the truth of a higher power to help in the fight against their illness, patients then visualize themselves donning this first piece of armor, the Belt of Truth, as a reward for their efforts and a sign of their commitment to fight the good fight.

Step 3: Submission

Once we identified a spiritual power greater than ourselves, we decided to turn our will and our lives over to the care of God as we understood him.

Understanding the Human Will

The concept of human will is thought to be one of the components of the soul of an individual. I will briefly describe several schools of thought on the subject that I think are relevant.

First, Judeo-Christian theology posits that humans are born with a will that is bent away from God and toward self. The three main enemies of humanity—the world, the flesh, and the Devil—conspire to bend our will to strive for experiences that bring us pleasure, to acquire possessions and monetary wealth, and to garner accomplishments and accolades (what Scripture calls "the lust of the flesh, the lust of the eyes, and the pride of life"[15]). However, for humans responsible to their higher power and benevolent taskmaster, pleasure is not the goal of life but rather the consequence of leading a morally pure life submitted to God's will.

While it is clear to believers that humans are not here to merely enjoy themselves, joy can indeed be achieved even in circumstances that have no possibility of pleasure, such as emotional or physical suffering. Joy, therefore, is an intentional emotion that is always directed toward an object, such as one's identified higher power. This is in contrast to pleasure, which is a conditional emotion wholly contingent upon circumstances.[16]

Historical Views on Will and Meaning

Friedrich Nietzsche, the renowned nineteenth-century German philosopher, introduced the concept of the "will to power." Nietzsche made a break with conventional notions of morality based on altruism and self-sacrifice by asserting that power dynamics and individual self-assertion underlie all human behavior, because the will to power is the fundamental drive inherent in all living beings. According to Nietzsche, the will to power incorporated the individual's quest for self-realization, mastery, and the actualization of one's potential. Unfortunately, his philosophical ideas were later hijacked by the German Nazi Party, who used them to justify authoritarianism, exploitation, and social Darwinism. In its extreme caricature, then, the will to power can and has been used to justify the striving for position and prominence over others. The Apostle John called this perversion of the human will "the pride of life."[17]

Historically noteworthy psychiatrists have also offered unique perspectives on the concept of human will in the common interest of understanding the motivations and inner workings of human behavior. Sigmund Freud's concept of will is embedded within his psychoanalytic theory, which suggests that both unconscious drives and internal psychological conflicts—largely outside of conscious awareness—shape human behavior. He proposed that humans are driven by instinctual forces, such as the sexual instincts (Eros) and the death drive (Thanatos), which often conflict with societal norms and moral values. For Freud, the actions of humans are often influenced by hidden motives and desires, leading to a sense of psychological determinism with minimal personal agency. The Apostle John called the bent of the will toward our instinctual drives and away from God "the lust of the flesh."[18]

Alfred Adler, a contemporary of Freud, also had views on the concept of will, though they differed somewhat from those of Freud. Adler's concept of will rested upon his belief that individuals are primarily motivated by the pursuit of meaning and purpose in their lives rather than by the pursuit of pleasure or power. Central to Adler's theory is the concept of "social interest," which refers to the individual's innate inclination to contribute to the welfare of others and society as a whole. Adler viewed social connectedness and cooperation as essential for psychological health and fulfillment.

Viktor Frankl's views on the concept of will are deeply intertwined with his existential philosophy and his personal experiences in several Nazi concentration camps during World War II. Unlike Freud's pleasure principle or Adler's will to meaning, Frankl's concept of will is closely linked to the existential struggle to find significance and value in one's existence, especially in the face of suffering and adversity. As mentioned earlier, Frankl emphasized the freedom of will, asserting that individuals have the capacity to choose their attitudes and responses to life's challenges, regardless of external circumstances. Frankl's emphasis on the existential dimension of meaning distinguishes his approach from Adler's more social and community-oriented perspective. For Frankl, meaning is deeply personal and subjective, arising from the individual's unique experiences, values, and aspirations.

More recently, Gerald May made a distinction between willfulness and willingness. May views willingness as a quality of openness, surrender, and acceptance of whatever life might throw at an individual, while embracing both joy and suffering as opportunities for growth and learning. In contrast, willfulness is characterized by a more rigid insistence on having things go according to one's own desires and preferences, often evidenced by a tendency to exert control over circumstances. Willfulness often arises from fear, insecurity, or a need for control, and May asserts that this needs to be relinquished in order to cultivate willingness as a pathway to spiritual growth.

The Will to Other: A New Paradigm

Ruachiatry puts forth the concept of "the will to other," in which autonomous individuals freely decide to relinquish control to their identified higher power. In this paradigm, patients do so in an attempt to be obedient to the two greatest commandments given by God: to love God and to love other people. This highest form of love is called *agape* in Greek, and it is characterized by a deliberate choice to selflessly submit one's will to serve another. This distinguishes it from other Greek words for love: *eros* (romantic passion), *philia* (brotherly friendship), and *storge* (instinctive familial affection). Individuals retain their unique and distinct will but choose to attempt to make the world a better place by serving others, enriching themselves by experiencing relationships with others, and accepting suffering allowed by the ultimate Other, with strength, dignity, and hope due to their faith in this Other. It is my opinion that this is the holy grail of spiritual health.

Reframing Submission as Strength

Submission has come to have a negative connotation in Western culture, because we erroneously believe the term implies an act being imposed against our will by an outside dominant force. Especially in the United States, we have come to value individual freedoms, rights, and autonomy to such a high degree that the term *submission* has become abhorrent. Most people probably envision a vanquished foe groveling for mercy at the feet of the victor in battle.

However, submission can be a voluntary act of free will by one who recognizes the greater power and authority of a benevolent other. Close but imperfect examples in our physical world include children voluntarily submitting to loving parents and citizens voluntarily submitting to a just and democratic government. Nevertheless, it is difficult for most people to completely and unquestionably submit to such earthly authority, because there is no such thing as a perfect parent or government.

In the spiritual realm, however, submission should be a more reasonable consideration if the patients' concept of their higher power is both benevolent and powerful. Submission is, in fact, such an important concept that it is the very foundation of the world's second most widely practiced religion, Islam, whose very name is derived from the Arabic root word *as-lama*, which means submission. Likewise, in Buddhism, *anatta* (no self) involves letting go of ego to align with universal truth, and in Hinduism, *bhakti yoga* (devotional surrender) encourages offering oneself to the divine. In Judaism, submission is less about annihilation of will and more about partnering with God through obedience and faith.

Recognizing who God is was the key to Step 2, but recognizing who God is *not* is the first task of Step 3. Patients must deduce that since there is a higher power, it is not they themselves. This makes intellectual sense, but the reality is that anytime we consider God's will for us—via the leading of his Spirit, his written expression in Scripture, or our moral compass, the conscience—and then decide to follow our own will instead, we are playing God. This is such a grievous crime against the Almighty that it is the first prohibition of the Ten Commandments God gave to Moses on Mount Sinai: "Thou shall have no other gods before me."[19]

Having come to the conclusion that there is, in fact, a God and it is not they themselves, patients must then decide whether or not to submit their will and life over to God, and if so, to what extent. As we have discussed earlier, humans are born with a non-functional dead spirit and with an inherited selfish will, which is bent away from God. This is why the founder of the world's largest religious faith, Jesus of Nazareth, taught that the two greatest commandments are to love the Lord your God supremely with all your being and to love your neighbor as yourself.[20] Jesus knew that we would love ourselves due to our inherently selfish nature and that it would take effort and intentionality for us to love God more than ourselves and even to love other people to the same degree that we love ourselves.

But Jesus did not merely espouse loving God and others. He exemplified both in his life by denying himself, submitting his will to God's, and serving others. And he taught that anyone desiring to follow him must do the same.[21] Jesus modeled what this looks like when he cried out in the garden of Gethsemane the night prior to his execution, "Father, if you are willing, please take this cup of suffering away from me. Yet, I want your will to be done, not mine."[22] In his humanity, Jesus understandably did not want to suffer the atrocities he would face on the Roman cross. However, he understood his mission, and despite the agony he knew he'd face, he voluntarily chose to submit his will to God's.[23] This is why, in the most famous prayer he taught to his followers,

Jesus asked them to pray that God's will, not their own will, be done on earth as it is in heaven.[24]

Jesus's voluntary submission of his will to God's will stands in stark contrast to Satan's rebellious will, as evidenced by his five "I will" statements recounted by the prophet Isaiah.

> *For you have said in your heart:*
> *"I will ascend into heaven,*
> *I will exalt my throne above the stars of God;*
> *I will also sit on the mount of the congregation*
> *On the farthest sides of the north.*
> *I will ascend above the heights of the clouds;*
> *I will be like the Most High."*[25]

It is important to notice that Satan did not announce his plans out loud. He thought they were secretly hidden within his heart, but God is omniscient and knows the secrets of our hearts.[26] Satan's pride and arrogance led him to aspire to five things reserved for the Most High God alone: the highest heavenly position, the rights of royalty both in heaven and on earth, attaining earthly position reserved for the Messiah, and achieving both the glory and likeness of God. It is a reminder that self-will, exalted above God's will, is always discovered by an omniscient God and eventually punished.

Finding Peace Through Surrender

Physicians must appreciate that deciding to abandon one's will for God's will and turning one's life over to his care are difficult and take a leap of faith. It entails essentially taking your hands off the steering wheel of your life and relinquishing control of your very soul to a God you cannot see. But it is somewhat easier if the higher power patients have identified in their earnest search is both benevolent and powerful. Patients must believe that, if they will only surrender, God will do for them in their illness what they are not able to do for themselves.

Working through Step 3 allows patients to simultaneously achieve peace with the first two of their seven enemies we discussed in Chapter 6—themselves and God. From there, two things occur simultaneously to enable patients to usher in a new life permeated with peace. Christians believe that if patients identify Jesus as their higher power and accept his substitutionary, sacrificial death on the cross as payment for their sin debt to God, then God the Father will send his Holy Spirit to replace patients' dead spirits. This Holy Spirit, in turn, empowers a new life in which the soul can indeed voluntarily come under the control of a benevolent, indwelling Spirit where there was once none. Furthermore, surrender of patients' wills to God's will pleases God so much that he grants them access to the second piece of spiritual armor needed to fight their spiritual battles—the Shoes of Peace.[27]

These shoes of the Roman soldier, called *caligae*, were a very sturdy hard leather shoe with iron hobnails embedded in the sole to enable soldiers to stand firm on the battlefield. In addition to facilitating patients to stand firm, the Shoes of Peace also enable patients to go on the offensive and advance against "the gates of hell."[28] With this peace, patients can now be confident in the midst of their suffering, knowing that, whatever the outcome, the all-powerful God is on their side and that "if God is for us, who can be against us?"[29]

Sometimes suffering is inevitable, and the only way out is through. But in the midst of their medical or psychological suffering, patients can now cling to the comforting truths that God never leaves us,[30] and in fact, he walks through the valley of the shadow of death with us.[31] If God, as the patient understands him, is omnipotent, he will ultimately win the war despite occasional losses of battles along the way. Furthermore, Scripture assures patients that

God will protect believers from evil spiritual forces as they walk through this world donned in their Shoes of Peace.[32]

The Apostle Paul's struggles with an unknown physical malady he called his "thorn in the flesh" provide an appropriate object lesson for patients suffering today. Paul states in his letter to the first-century church in Corinth, a Greek city-state, that he was snatched away from earth and given the privilege of going to the highest heaven, where he received "such wonderful revelations from God."[33] Some scholars believe this may be a first-century account of what physicians now call a near-death experience from fourteen years earlier, when he was stoned while preaching in the city of Derbe, in Asia Minor, and then dragged outside the city gates and left for dead.

Paul goes on to describe the reasons he believes he struggles with a chronic, severe physical malady despite his great faith:

> So, to keep me from becoming proud, I was given a thorn in my flesh, a messenger from Satan to torment me. . . . Three different times I begged the Lord to take it away. Each time he said, "My grace is all you need. My power works best in weakness." So now I am glad to boast about my weaknesses, so that the power of Christ can work through me. That's why I take pleasure in my weaknesses, and in the insults, hardships, persecutions, and troubles that I suffer for Christ. For when I am weak, then I am strong.[34]

Essentially, God allowed Satan to torment Paul with this physical malady for a reason—to keep him humble. Paul clearly identifies Satan as his tormentor, the one who brings sickness to Paul's body. It seemed as though Satan was winning, getting his way by afflicting Paul. Understandably, Paul did not like this and resorted to begging God to intervene on his behalf and cure him as he knew only God could. God, however, reminded Paul that God is sovereign and that there is purpose to the suffering he permits in our lives. Generally speaking, it is my belief that the greater the unjustified suffering (that is, suffering not due to negligence or unwise life decisions on the part of the sufferer), the greater God's call on one's life.

Paul responded rightly to his unjustified suffering through surrender to God's will. But Paul's ability to find joy and peace in the midst of his suffering is clearly God's power working through Paul's weakness.[35] This joy and peace is only made possible by Paul's acceptance of and submission to God's will for him to suffer physical infirmity. Remembering that "God works all things together for the good of those who love him, who are called according to his purpose,"[36] this very same joy and peace are also available today to patients like you and me.

But in order to find this joy, peace, and strength in the midst of suffering medical or mental illness, patients must submit their will and their life to their higher power. As the great Methodist preacher and evangelist John Wesley once said, "Let each one in all things deny his or her own will, however pleasing, and do the will of God, however painful."[37] This surrender to God's will exemplifies that living faith in which patients' beliefs are completely aligned with their actions.[38] In fact, submission to God's will carries eternal significance, as stated by Jesus: "Not everyone . . . will enter the Kingdom of Heaven. Only those who actually do the will of my Father in heaven will enter."[39]

Patients must, therefore, resolve to submit to God's will in order to have a more abundant, victorious life over difficulties, such as illness, in their short time on earth as well as to have eternal life that will one day be free from all sickness, pain, and even death itself. Until then, patients can come to learn that in the context of eternity, their medical afflictions are indeed light and momentary and serve God's greater purpose of working out the patients' "eternal weight of glory"—an everlasting future reward for responding in faith to temporary suffering now.[40] Only the life built upon the solid foundation of submitting to and actually doing God's will can withstand the floods of affliction, when the storms of life inevitably come.

This surrender does not eliminate the struggle but reframes it as part of a larger spiritual narrative, where the patient becomes a co-warrior with their higher power against the unseen forces of illness. It is a courageous act, requiring humility and faith, and it sets the stage for the radical renovation described in the next chapter.

14

STEPS 4–9: RADICAL RENOVATION

The middle phase of the Ruachiatry journey—Steps 4 to 9—marks a period of radical renovation, where patients actively dismantle the spiritual strongholds that contribute to their illness and rebuild their lives on a foundation of faith.

Step 4: Traumas and Lies

We made a list of circumstances, individuals, or groups that had harmed us, what they had done, and the subsequent lies we had believed about ourselves.

Due to the invisible war that many patients were previously unaware of, physicians ought to help them recognize that they may have heart wounds with which they have never dealt. Neglected wounds worsen over time, and our spiritual enemies likely use these wounds as an opportunity to lay in patients' minds a firm foundation of lies upon which the enemies can build strongholds.

Step 4 in Ruachiatry is to begin to clean house. In my work in the field of psychiatry, I have found that often, patients who have experienced trauma will in essence banish all associated memories and feelings to the proverbial cellar in their mind, locking the door behind it. Repression of the associated hurtful feelings and justifiable anger often leads to resentment and eventually bitterness—an open-door invitation for unseen malevolent entities to gain access to their minds and hearts and start building a fortress to inhabit. Cleaning house involves unlocking the cellar door and dealing with what is down there, putting it to rest once and for all, and securing all open doors to our spiritual house.

Traumas: Uppercase *T* vs. Lowercase *t*

Before their spiritual awakening, patients had a nonfunctional dead spirit within them and no effective armor to protect them from heart wounds. Spiritual foes took advantage and influenced others to emotionally wound patients. We all have experienced traumatic events in the course of our lives, some of which are traumas with a lowercase *t* and some with an uppercase *T*. For example, most uppercase-*T* traumas are relatively rare and are well known to lead to physical or emotional problems, albeit to varying degrees. Examples include compound bone fractures, large surface area burns, rape, natural disasters, dangerous combat, and witnessing heinous violent crimes or unexpected death, to name only a few. But even with these uppercase-*T* traumas, there is some variability in the degree to which they negatively affect individual patients. Research and experience show that it is not so much the actual event that defines a trauma's ultimate effect but one's reaction to it.

Lowercase-*t* traumas, on the other hand, are ubiquitous and tend to be in the eye of the beholder, meaning that what one patient considers a traumatic event may not be experienced as traumatic at all by another patient. One of the reasons for this is the concept of *resilience*, thought to be a complex combination of both innate and learned coping. Factors known to be predictive of improved coping with trauma include 1) good problem-solving capabilities, 2) the ability to regulate emotions effectively, 3) persistent, realistic optimism, and 4) a strong social support network.

While some traumas are clearly accidents, so-called acts of God, or acts of war, many of patients' traumas are caused by other people they encounter in their everyday lives. In Step 4, the clinician asks patients to recognize that they likely have heart wounds due to experiences they construe as traumatic, be they uppercase-*T* or lowercase-*t* traumas, by making an exhaustive list going back to childhood.

Cataloging Past Hurts

Next, the clinician asks patients to briefly describe what happened and then whether they believe the hurt was inflicted intentionally or unintentionally. Just as in criminal law, it is important to examine the *mens rea* (mental state and intent) of the perpetrators of their traumas, because some traumas are intentional in nature and some are not, perhaps being due to ignorance, neglect, or accident. I have found that, in general, it is much easier for patients to forgive wounds that they recognize as unintentional or accidental.

Demolishing Strongholds: Replacing Lies with the Truth

Next comes the all-important step of tearing down strongholds, those demonic citadels in patients' minds that were built upon a foundation of lies from wounding messengers. If patients can destroy the foundation, the walls will inevitably come tumbling down. There's an old saying that if you give the Devil a toehold, it will soon become his foothold, and then eventually a stronghold. I like to think of strongholds as dwelling places our spiritual enemies have built from which they conduct their ongoing business of reinforcing the lies that allowed them into patients' minds in the first place. The walls of these evil fortresses are built with harmful thought patterns, negative attitudes, and hurtful messages from the outside world. In Step 4, patients must tear down mental and emotional strongholds and permanently evict their malevolent inhabitants.

Here, especially, is where patients must recognize that the weapons they have are not physical but spiritual, having, according to Scripture, "divine power to demolish strongholds."[1] To do so, they must first identify the lies they have believed due to their heart wounds and then replace the lies with the truth according to their identified higher power. This truth can often be grasped by means of the writings considered holy scripture in patients' identified religion.

Armor to Protect the Heart

The armor to be taken up at the conclusion of this step is the Breastplate of Righteousness. This piece of armor obviously protects the heart, and since the patients have at this point started to heal from their past heart wounds, it is imperative that they now put on this piece of armor to protect their heart in the future. Many patients have suffered heart wounds in the past because they were not even aware they were in a war and needed to defend themselves. Things will be very different moving forward.

The Breastplate of Righteousness not only protects the heart but also allows patients to endure with joy whatever malice God's will allows other people or demons to inflict. But patients must remain vigilant and committed to working on their purity in all their thoughts, conduct, and conversations. Impurity causes cracks in the armor, and Satan knows exactly where to find it and send in precision-guided fiery missiles to re-wound their hearts. Righteousness and purity, on the other hand, will make patients as bold as a lion, despite their suffering.[2]

Following is a suggested template to function as a worksheet for both Step 4 and the upcoming Step 5:

Worksheet: Inventory of Traumas Suffered

Who hurt you?	What did they do?	Was it intentional or unintentional?	Lies I believed as a result of my hurt	Truth according to my higher power	Degree of current resentment (0–10)	Asked God for the strength to forgive? (Yes or No)

Step 5: Choosing Forgiveness

We ranked the degree of resentment and bitterness we still harbor and asked God to give us the strength to forgive those who hurt us, be they individuals, groups, or institutions.

Measuring Resentment's Toll

Having completed the difficult task of identifying past hurts, what happened, judging whether it was intentional or unintentional, identifying the lying packages they received and believed, and replacing the strongholds of lies with the truth from their identified higher power, patients' task in Step 5 is to examine how all of these have affected them emotionally and then to seek to forgive with the help of their higher power. The initial task of Step 5 is for patients to rank the current degree of their resentment, and since resentment takes time to build, patients need to gain an understanding of how the resentment came about and evolved over time into its current state.

Understanding Anger's Roots

Defining some common associated terms at this point is important, so let's start with the emotion of *anger*—a normal emotion that is disconcerting and frightening to many patients. Emotions, including anger, are not inherently bad in and of themselves, but as the shallowest part of our soul, they must be controlled. Emotions should not be allowed to drive the bus, so to speak, because emotionally uncontrolled drivers tend to cause wrecks.

Anger, although common and often understandable based on the circumstances, most often carries a negative connotation. It is a potentially dangerous emotion, having the power to enslave. "Anyone who can make you angry," said the Greek Stoic philosopher Epictetus, "becomes your master."[3]

Anger arises in reaction to one of three circumstances. The first common and ubiquitous antecedent of the emotion of anger is frustration and irritation in reaction to one's needs, wants, or expectations not being met. These often require no forgiveness on the patient's part since they tend to be petty annoyances born of happenstance and are common to everyday life. Therefore, they should be expected, and patients should decide ahead of time how they are going to respond to these frequent irritants, making it less likely they will react.

The main difference between responding and reacting is that responding entails utilizing one's cognitive faculties to decide in advance how to address a foreseeable problem, whereas reacting is a quick, typically emotional, way of handling frustration. If patients have difficulty handling irritations that are a normal part of life, they are likely to have even greater difficulty handling the other two precursors of anger, namely being hurt physically or emotionally and being treated in a fashion they consider to be unjust or unfair.

Because both expressed and repressed anger can be very destructive forces, how one deals with them is of great importance. Anger will inevitably come, but it must be managed appropriately; otherwise, it may become a grievous sin akin to murder itself. John Wesley, the founder of the Methodist Christian denomination, defined anger as "the first rising of disgust at those who injure you, opposite to forgiving."[4] This small fire can either be kindled or snuffed out quickly. Anger is best dealt with immediately, because small controllable fires can become huge, destructive wildfires over time if neglected. What could have been extinguished with a small amount of water or a stamping of the foot becomes a raging force necessitating huge amounts of water delivered via both ground and air efforts in order to exterminate it.

Most religious traditions espouse that anger is nearly always bad unless it manifests as righteous indignation, a justified anger in which one is defending another person who is being attacked unjustly and harshly. The example from Christian tradition involves Jesus, who despite being treated unjustly many times, according to Scripture, bears no record of becoming angry or attempting to defend himself— even upon being unjustly condemned to execution on a Roman cross.[5] Jesus became angry only when God's name, reputation, or house of worship was denigrated in some way. One such time is described in Scripture when Jesus overturned money changers' tables in the court- yard of the Temple of Jerusalem and then fashioned a whip of cords to drive out animals that merchants were selling there. He performed these acts because he believed the merchants and money changers were turning the temple into a "den of thieves."[6] Jesus's defense of his Father's name, reputation, and place of worship was an act of righ- teous indignation, not unbridled anger resulting from personal injury, frustration, or common irritation.

Holding on to anger and not discharging it appropriately from the very start predictably leads to an increasingly larger fire that can turn deadly. Psychologically, this progression occurs in the fol- lowing fashion: Someone is frustrated, hurt, or treated unfairly, leading to an understandable spark of anger. Figuratively speaking, when the spark lands on a dry, unwatered portion of their mind, a small fire is ignited. If untended, the spark of anger in the mind grows over time into a blazing inferno, becoming resentment. The word *resentment* has its origins in the prefix *re-*, meaning "again," and the Latin verb *sentire*, meaning "to feel." Hence, resentment is a state of voluntarily choosing to feel the pain from the origi- nal wounding again and again, allowing the small fire to continue to grow. Patients' focus needs to change from old pain to new strength drawn from their higher power.

Unresolved resentment gives way, eventually, to bitterness, a state of settled anger analogous to a deadly weed whose root runs deep, making it difficult to kill once entrenched in the soil of one's mind. Old Testament Hebrew uses the term *bitter* to describe poison, and Scripture states that this poisonous root inevitably leads to trouble and defilement of many people besides just the one harboring bitterness.[7] This is the truth behind the saying "hurt people hurt people." Patients must recognize that their choice to recurrently experience the same pain of the initial injury is simply madness, a severe mental malady that will lead them to metaphorically ingest a poisonous root, severely harming themselves and others in the process. The Apostle Paul, the author of the majority of the New Testament, prescribes the remedy for this grave situation in his letter to the first-century church in Ephesus:

Get rid of all bitterness, rage and anger, brawling and slander, along with every form of malice. Be kind and compassionate to one another, forgiving each other, just as, in Christ, God forgave you.[8]

Rage or wrath are outward manifestations of anger that usually present as sudden outbursts out of proportion to the supposed antecedent. Wrath arises from lasting displeasure that creates an environment in the heart that is ready to explode whenever a small amount of irritant, frustration, or reminder of a past hurt presents itself and acts as an accelerant, predictably leading to an explosion. The wise King Solomon of ancient Israel recognized the importance of controlling your temper when he insisted, "Anger labels you a fool."[9]

In contrast to the outward actions seen in rage, the progression of anger to its final phase of malice concerns the inner attitudes and intentions of the heart, which patients must guard above all else.[10] Patients must be increasingly concerned with their internal motives, not merely the external control of their reactions to hurt or injustice. Even though affected patients may never actually murder someone, their unresolved anger may eventually grow into malice, defined by the *Oxford English Dictionary* as "the intention or desire to do evil," legally known as the prerequisite state of mind behind murder.

Patients' self-righteousness must be challenged, and they must come to the realization that things they thought were of little consequence, such as anger, calling other people names, and attacking other people's character, will bring about the same degree of punishment as murder in the eyes of God.[11] This is the rationale behind Step 5 requiring patients to honestly assess the degree to which they still harbor resentment or bitterness toward those people or institutions who hurt them. By ranking their degree on a scale of 0 to 10, patients can see how much inner work needs to be done to metaphorically dig up each root of bitterness that has caused trouble.

From Bitterness to Freedom

Once identified, how exactly do patients go about the task of getting rid of resentment, bitterness, wrath, or malice once and for all? The answer is simple but far from easy—forgiveness.

But forgiveness does not imply granting trust and reconciliation to the perpetrator of hurt or injustice; those must be earned over time by the efforts of the perpetrator. I have heard it said that we are never more like God than when we are forgiving, especially of one who is undeserving, as that gives us the opportunity to display grace. The reasoning behind the axiom "to err is human but to forgive is divine" is that forgiveness is so difficult in practice for mere mortals that it requires the help of a higher power. Hopefully, by means of Step 2, patients have identified their ultimate higher power and can turn to him for help.

Just as patients discovered earlier that there is a higher power and that they are not it, here patients must appreciate that their higher power is the one and only legitimate judge, who sees all, including the state of each individual's heart, and is by nature loving, righteous, and just. Ultimately, God is the only being with the ability to judge fairly. It is completely understandable that patients desire justice, but they must resist the urge to act as judge and condemn or sentence the perpetrator, because there is only one judge, and we are not him.

Trusting Divine Justice

Whether or not patients acknowledge Jesus as God's Son, most admit that Jesus was a very wise and honorable teacher, whose example with regard to handling unjust suffering is worth emulating. As Scripture recounts:

> *He did not retaliate when he was insulted, nor threaten revenge when he suffered. He left his case in the hands of God, who always judges fairly.*[12]

If possible and appropriate, a patient can be encouraged to arrange a private meeting with their perpetrator and explain how his or her actions hurt the patient. Admittedly, there are times when this is neither safe nor advisable. If when the perpetrator is gently, privately confronted, he or she listens, expresses remorse, and apologizes, the patient is on the way to restoring the relationship. But what should clinicians recommend if this repentance does not occur because a debt remains that the perpetrator must pay?

Since the patient is not authorized to extract payment, it seems as though justice will not be satisfied. Here is where the all-important step comes into play of trusting one's higher power to eventually settle the debt and exact justice. This is described in Scripture:

Beloved, never avenge yourselves, but leave the way open for God's wrath [and his judicial righteousness]; for it is written, "Vengeance is Mine, I will repay," says the Lord.[13]

Don't say, "I will get even for this wrong." Wait for the Lord to handle the matter.[14]

Revenge harms one's own soul, and the patient releasing the debt to God sets two captives free—both the debtor and the one owed recompense, who willingly and foolishly may have been reliving the pain again and again. Forgiveness is the only way to let go of the anger aimed at the perpetrator of hurt or injustice. It is therefore vital that we accept that we have no right to withhold forgiveness from others, since God himself has graciously granted us unmerited forgiveness.[15] Jesus warns how God deals with those who refuse to forgive others their relatively small debt in comparison to how God has forgiven us:

Then the king called in the man he had forgiven and said, "You evil servant! I forgave you that tremendous debt because you pleaded with me. Shouldn't you have mercy on your fellow servant, just as I had mercy on you?" Then the angry king sent the man to prison to be tortured until he had paid his entire debt. That's what my heavenly Father will do to you if you refuse to forgive your brothers and sisters from your heart.[16]

Whether patients' anger sits at the surface or is buried deep inside, they must not avoid it, minimize it, rationalize it, or feed it. They must face it head-on, allowing the reality of the grave consequences if they choose otherwise to compel them to ask God for the divine strength to forgive those who have hurt them. Healthcare providers ought to always call upon patients to represent their higher self through the highest form of the four loves—*agape*—which is said by the Apostle Paul to keep no record of wrongs.[17] This is why the prosperous and wise King Solomon of ancient Israel once wrote "Love prospers when a fault is forgiven, but dwelling on it separates close friends."[18] Adding forgiveness to patients' new path of acceptance, commitment, humility, submission to God's will, and peace will enable them to not only gain a better cognitive understanding of God but also experience the forgiveness that only he can and will give, if it's sought.

Step 6: Traumas We Inflicted upon Others

We made a list of all people we have harmed and admitted to God, ourselves, and to another human being the exact nature of our wrongs.

Following is a suggested template to function as a Step 6 worksheet:

Worksheet: Inventory of Traumas Inflicted

Whom did you hurt?	What did you do?	Was it intentional or unintentional?	What could you have done instead?	What was the nature of your character defect(s) involved?	Have you forgiven yourself? (Yes or No)	Admitted to God & another person the nature of your wrongs? (Yes or No)

Reflecting on Harms We Inflicted

As discussed in Step 5, patients suffering from illness, like me and all other humans since the dawn of time, are hurt people, collateral damage in the unseen spiritual war between God and rebellious spiritual beings. And since hurt people hurt people, Step 6 is the place for patients to examine and admit—first to themselves, then to God and another person—the people they have hurt and exactly what they did to those people. Hurting other humans, the pinnacle of creation made in the image of God himself, is a grievous miscarriage of justice, what many faiths call *sin*, meaning missing the mark. God takes it very seriously and so should we.

The first question, "Whom did you hurt?", should go back to childhood. This need not involve minor infractions that are common but rather the more serious ones that may have had a more lasting negative effect on the recipients of the hurtful behavior. Next, patients should identify whether their infraction was intentional, as accidental or even negligent infractions are usually easier to deal with from a psychological standpoint. The fourth column addresses what patients could have done differently. Exploring this is important to help patients see that there were likely other better options, and thus, this exercise could help them respond differently in the future when faced with a similar circumstance. Psychologically, this helps empower patients to know that they have learned from their mistakes and that the same transgression is less likely to occur in the future.

Analyzing Character Flaws

Column 5 concerns character defects, as patients often come to see a pattern emerge in the treatment of people they have hurt. Here, patients explore whether they were selfish, dishonest, prideful, arrogant, jealous, suspicious, resentful, bitter, impatient, fearful, or merely inconsiderate. These are common examples of character defects, but this list is far from exhaustive. Again, recognizing these patterns can serve the same purpose as asking patients what they could have done differently. Admitting character defects is patients' first step toward empowering themselves to make positive changes. Sometimes, character defects are many years in the making, and so these deeply entrenched patterns of thinking and behavior may need to be addressed with the help of a competent psychotherapist. Healthcare providers should discuss this briefly with their patients, explain that these uncovered character defects may be an impediment to psychological and spiritual wellness, and make a referral if patients are willing.

Seeking Self-Forgiveness

Column 6 asks patients if they have forgiven themselves. After exploring in detail and taking responsibility for their role in these hurts, patients are often able to start forgiving themselves if they have not done so previously. As discussed in Step 5, Jesus insinuated that patients have no right to withhold forgiveness from any human, including themselves, because of the degree to which they have been forgiven by God. Again, if a patient gets stuck in this area, a healthcare provider may need to refer him or her to a psychotherapist to work through it.

Confessing to Heal

The final phase of this stage involves patients admitting their hurtful transgressions against others to God and another person whom they trust to be nonjudgmental (this could be the clinician). This task may be somewhat faster for faithful Roman Catholics who have been observing the sacrament of confession regularly, because they have already confessed their wrongs to God and a priest. The rationale behind this last phase lies in the Scriptural promise that if patients confess their wrongdoings against others, God will be true to his own just nature and faithfully respond by forgiving their trespasses and cleansing them of all unrighteous thoughts, desires, and deeds.[19] God, once again, can and will do for patients what they are not able to do for themselves, if patients respond in the right fashion with humility, honesty, and submission to God's will.

Step 7: Amends

We became willing to make amends to people we had harmed and then made direct amends to such people wherever possible and appropriate.

Embracing Reconciliation

Initiating steps toward reconciliation is the goal of Step 7. First, it involves the will, providing yet another opportunity for patients to act in humility and voluntarily submit their will to that of their higher power. Patients can be confident that reconciliation is always God's will, because, as chronicled earlier, God, who was formerly one of mankind's seven enemies, initiated reconciliation with mankind, bringing us peace. So patients, by initiating reconciliation with people they have hurt, again have the wonderful opportunity of being able to act in a fashion similar to that of their higher power. In Judaism, reconciliation is fulfilled through *shuv* (returning to others with amends), in Islam through *sadaqah* (charity) to heal past wrongs, in Buddhism through *dana* (generosity) to others, and in Hinduism through *karma yoga* (selfless action) to balance past actions.

This reconciliation process is accomplished by means of amends—doing something to correct a mistake or a bad situation that one has caused. When patients become willing to make amends, they have made a decision to go further than merely apologizing for their transgression. They accept full responsibility for their part, acknowledging their wrongs. This next step is crucial because it is commanded by God in Scripture, and failure to follow it hinders patients' connection with their higher power. Jesus discussed this very issue in his famous Sermon on the Mount:

> *Therefore, if you are offering your gift at the altar and there remember that your brother or sister has something against you, leave your gift there in front of the altar. First go and be reconciled to them; then come and offer your gift.*[20]

Acting with Courage

God desires one's obedience rather than any gift or sacrifice we humans can offer.[21] Hence, obeying his will regarding reconciliation is the essential precursor to the second part of Step 7—actually taking action in an effort to make up for what has happened in the past. At this point, patients are advised to contact the people they have wronged, but this is not always possible or advisable. For example, contact may not be possible if people have died, moved, or if their contact information is not readily available on the internet. Also, there may be circumstances in which contact could put the patient at risk of violence or legal action. For the other persons on the list, it is recommended that prior to meeting or talking with them, patients should ponder how they can make up for the past. If patients cannot think of an appropriate amend, after offering a formal apology, they should ask the offended party, "Is there anything I can do to make it up to you?"

If the offended party says there is not, it is wise for patients to extend some act of appreciation anyway, such as sending them a note with a small gift, stating that they appreciate their willingness to meet.

Step 8: From Fear to Faith

We made a list of things we fear and consciously chose to cast our cares upon God, having faith that he is both willing and able to help those who humbly seek him.

Confronting a Fearful Age

The times in which we live have been called the age of anxiety, and as a psychiatrist, I commonly evaluate and treat patients suffering from anxiety disorders. With economic volatility, political polarization, climate change, pandemics, threats of nuclear annihilation, and the rapid changes globally due to the accelerated pace and proliferation of technological advances, we have a degree of insecurity in the world today that is unparalleled in all of history. It's a perfect recipe for concern and worry. Additionally, the twenty-four-hour news cycle, social media, and the internet enable bad news to be accessible instantaneously to almost everyone on the planet. The sinister powers behind the running of this world system know well that it is much easier to control a fearful populace, which will be primed to accept measures offered by its government to increase perceived safety and security, even at the expense of voluntarily sacrificing some of its freedoms. "Never let a good crisis go to waste," first uttered by Winston Churchill in the midst of World War II, seems to be the motto that our unseen enemies use either to take advantage of or to manufacture a crisis in order to better control the masses. We thought technology would bring us increased productivity and more leisure time, only to find, like most of the Devil's deceptions, that was half true. It came with the hidden costs of increased stress and fear as well as enslavement to the dopamine hits always available via social media.

Nothing steals one's joy and peace of mind as much as chronic worries, anxiety, and fear, in my opinion. The real travesty is that patients are putting a down payment on something they will likely never own. For example, a recent study of patients suffering from generalized anxiety disorder, which is characterized by long-standing uncontrollable worries, found that more than 91 percent of the things subjects worried about never came to fruition.[22] I believe we must expose and challenge the deceit behind these worries in order to truly help patients in their struggles with anxiety.

The cognitive aspects of anxiety often lead to predictable physical manifestations, such as arousal of the fight-or-flight autonomic nervous system, muscle tension, gastrointestinal distress, and insomnia, to name a few. So, how should patients fight fears that appear inevitable in the face of an uncertain and rapidly changing global environment?

Psychotherapy, particularly CBT, has proven beneficial for many patients. Furthermore, medications can be helpful for physiological manifestations of anxiety, better enabling patients to work on cognitive strategies and coping skills, once their hyperarousal is dampened. Medication alone is very rarely the remedy, however.

These psychological and medical treatments can be helpful, particularly in combination when appropriate. Nevertheless, I often find that patients continue to suffer some degree of residual symptoms, and the neglect of clinicians to address the spiritual component of anxiety may be one reason.

The Bible encourages its readers not to worry or have fear an astounding 365 times. It also supplies the remedy—faith. Much like forgiveness, it is simple but not easy. Ralph Waldo Emerson once rightly said, "Sorrow looks back, worry looks around, faith looks up."[23]

Sowing Seeds of Faith

Faith starts metaphorically with a tiny seed that is planted. The law of reaping and sowing says that human beings reap what we sow, more than we sow, later than we sow.[24] If we sow a tiny seed of faith, we will not reap grapes, olives, or anything else but faith, and a greater measure than we originally sowed. But it takes time. With each step of faith, patients draw closer to their higher power and see him move in their lives, further increasing their faith. And each of these small steps of faith cumulatively becomes a walk of faith. Without faith, it is impossible to please God, but faith is indeed attainable for those willing to seek him.[25] It takes the courage to take a step in the dark. But patients can be confident that their higher power is there to help them in their walk of faith.[26]

Here is where God supplies another piece of armor for patients to use in the spiritual warfare that affects their health—the Shield of Faith. This shield of a first-century Roman soldier was more like a door, a large rectangular shield called a *scutum*. In battle, soldiers could enter a formation called *testudo*, akin to a large tortoise shell, in which they would link their scuta together, forming a barrier that was impenetrable from the front and top. Alone, but especially in tandem, these shields provided soldiers with certainty of protection against the enemies' arrows. Similarly, the Shield of Faith that God supplies gives the certainty of total protection, because omnipotent God himself acts as the shield.[27]

When patients experience anxiety, I often ask them, "What's the worst thing that could happen?" Often, they give various answers, but I remind them that the worst thing is death. But Christianity teaches that Jesus defeated the Devil, who formerly held the power over death. Jesus then overcame death, which Scripture says, "set free all who have lived their lives as slaves to the fear of dying."[28] I encourage Christian patients by explaining that they no longer have to live as slaves to the fear of death, because whomever Jesus's sacrifice sets free is free indeed.[29]

When patients believe this and accept Jesus's sacrifice on their behalf, they can then put on the Helmet of Salvation to protect their minds from fear, knowing that even if they die, they will one day rise and be given a new, incorruptible body that will be impervious to death. Patients must cast down strongholds in their minds using their spiritual weapons. Spirits, malevolent enemies with a will all their own, must be cast out.[30] And behind much of the fear and deceitful worries that are not responsive to normally effective biological and psychological treatments may lie a spirit that is not from God but from our invisible enemy. Evidence of this is found in Scripture's assurances that God's Spirit grants patients love, power, and a sound mind and has not given patients who suffer from anxiety the spirit of fear.[31]

Because patients now have a new spirit to replace their dead spirit with which they were born, the Spirit of their higher power is now readily available to help.[32] But to appropriate this help, patients must first identify their specific fears and the reasons for them. They must take a look inward to discern what part of their self-will led to those fears. Was their self-esteem, financial or relationship security, ambition, or sexual confidence jostled?

Casting out the Spirit of Fear

Once fears have been exposed and their stronghold dwellings in patients' minds have been torn down, the lying spirits must now be evicted. The following step calls for patients to cast out their fear and the spirit behind it onto their higher power, as instructed in Step 3, completely trusting their lives to God's care.[33]

Following is a suggested template to function as a Step 8 worksheet:

Worksheet: Inventory of Fears

List of fears	Why are you fearful?	Part of self that caused the fear	Did you cast your cares upon your higher power?	Have you put on the Shield of Faith?	Have you put on the Helmet of Salvation?

Step 9: Vigilant and Sober

We made a decision to vigilantly guard our mind and to cease the use of any and all mind- or mood-altering substances unless prescribed by a physician.

Cleansing the Mind

After tearing down strongholds and casting out fears, patients can enjoy the benefit of a renewed mind. In Step 9, patients must pledge to be sober and vigilant in order to maintain a physical and mental environment that is clean and well protected, having no open doors to give their enemies further access.[34]

While sobriety is usually associated with the absence of mind-altering chemicals, in a more general sense, sobriety is a state of being in which one's mind is free from any influences outside of one's higher power. The enemies of the world, the flesh, and the Devil all offer intoxicating substitutes to fill the spiritual vacuum that is the result of our dead spirit. However, Scripture admonishes us to not become intoxicated with alcohol (or other drugs) but to be filled by the Spirit that is sent by God to guide us once we decide to turn our will and every aspect of our lives over to his care.[35] Only under complete influence of God's Spirit is there safety, joy, and power to handle adversity in life. Outside of this influence lurks dangers and calamity.

A brief sidenote: I fully appreciate that the vast majority of people can occasionally consume small amounts of alcohol responsibly without becoming intoxicated or without having any physical, relational, occupational, or legal problems whatsoever. However, as a physician, I can unequivocally state that with regard to one's overall health, it is better to abstain. This is especially true when patients are suffering from either physical or mental illness, a time they ought to be focusing on their recovery and therefore not consuming any mind- or mood-altering substance that could potentially hinder that.

Standing Watch Against Evil

Whereas sobriety is a state of being, vigilance is a state of action signifying a careful watch for danger. Patients need to live in constant awareness of the invisible war they are caught up in and their relentless and powerful spiritual enemies, who are seeking opportunities to gain access to their lives. The truth is that negative spiritual forces cannot take any ground in this war for human souls unless patients give it to them. Once patients become a dwelling place of the new, living Spirit from God, their bodies become a holy temple into which they must not allow the Devil a place.[36]

Patients must also be vigilant not to create a climate that makes the Devil feel welcome, because his toehold will become a foothold and inevitably another stronghold to replace the ones patients have labored so intensively to tear down. Wicked spiritual forces will retreat if patients resist them by standing firm, remaining sober and vigilant, and submitting their self-will to the will of their higher power.[37] But these spiritual enemies will look for opportunities to return if invited or given the right environment, and the latter state is often worse for patients than before the unseen enemy fled in the first place.[38]

In ancient times, guards standing watch served not only to keep out enemies but also to allow those with lawful rights to enter a palace or city. Likewise, keeping patients' minds aligned with their higher self, which is spiritually connected to God, takes more than just guarding the gates of entrance to the fortress of their minds. It also entails actively pursuing things that edify and fortify their minds.

Fortifying with Virtue

Clinicians should encourage their patients to actively fill their minds with whatever things are good and deserve praise: things that are true, noble, right, pure, lovely, and honorable.[39] Patients ought to abstain from watching, listening to, eating, drinking, or participating in anything that does not meet these criteria to avoid conforming again to the behavior and customs of the world system run by their powerful spiritual enemy.[40] Admittedly, this is increasingly difficult in a secular society that promotes sensuality, emotions, the priority of self, technology, and entertainment over spirituality, humility, and simplicity. Patients need support from their higher power to avoid such temptations. But a community of like-minded people, or at least an accountability partner, can be a tremendous addition for protecting the fortress of their minds and navigating this world system that is stacked against them.

15

STEPS 10–12: DRAWING CLOSER TO GOD

Draw near to God and he will draw near to you.

—JAMES 4:8 (NLT)

As a loving Father, God initiates the pursuit of his lost human children.[1] Once people enter into a relationship with God, he promises to never leave them nor forsake them.[2] But members of his human family will still leave God at times, either when distracted by the cares of this life or pursuing their self-will. Drawing closer to God will require intentionality, endurance, and persistence on the part of all patients.

The final three steps of Ruachiatry focus on patients making a conscious decision to draw close to their higher power by developing the daily discipline to actually carve out time from their busy schedules to hear from him. But since God historically has very rarely spoken audibly, how can patients hear from him today? Primarily through two means—reading holy scripture and personal prayer.[3]

Like all human beings, patients must realize that the only way to get to know and develop a relationship with God is to invest time with him. Because this is difficult in our busy, often hectic, twenty-first-century lives, this private one-on-one time must be planned, prioritized, and protected. The most effective soldiers for good in this spiritual war stand firm in obstinate continuance of the regular practice of spiritual disciplines, despite opposition.[4]

Step 10: Seeking Spiritual Wisdom

We made a decision to forgo or entirely relinquish any effort to gain spiritual understanding, knowledge, or wisdom apart from the orthodox teachings attributed to our higher power.

Rejecting Lesser Sources of Wisdom

In Step 10, patients decide to abandon all other means of obtaining spiritual insights, knowledge, and wisdom outside of the established and approved teachings of the religious faith of their higher power. If God is our high power, his holy scriptures are able to make us wise.[5] In Judaism, this aligns with Torah study, and Christians add to it the New Testament as the path to divine wisdom. In Islam, *'ilm* (knowledge) is sought through the Quran and Hadith. Buddhism emphasizes *prajna* (wisdom) through the dharma, and Hinduism values *jnana* (knowledge) gained from the Vedas and Upanishads.

Abandoning all other means includes patients' own vain human efforts, the efforts of others (regardless of how wise their philosophies and keen their intellects may appear to the rest of the world), and any supposedly esoteric spiritual knowledge or wisdom offered by occult sources. In our modern age, the Devil primarily employs three general attacks against ultimate truth: philosophy, the occult, and science.

The Limits of Human Philosophy

The first illegitimate means our spiritual enemy uses to divert humans from ultimate truth is through human philosophy, the love and pursuit of wisdom by human intellectual efforts. By this, I do not mean to imply that the academic branch of the humanities called *philosophy* is devoid of merit or inherently evil. On the contrary, many keen intellectual insights and truths can be gleaned from the academic study of philosophy. However, the Bible states that heavy reliance upon worldly wisdom is akin to building a home on a foundation of sand, and there are several fundamental problems with philosophy as a whole.

First, it is wisdom as defined by finite and sinful man, rather than from omniscient, holy God. Purportedly the wisest man in all of history, King Solomon of ancient Israel, "set out to learn everything," but ultimately came to learn firsthand that "pursuing all this is like chasing the wind." He then summed up the results of his quest. "Here is my final conclusion," he said, "Fear God and obey his commands, for this is everyone's duty."[6]

Furthermore, history itself shows that each subsequent generation has developed new schools of philosophical thought, but none of the truths on which they were built were fixed or permanent. Thus, there are numerous contradictory branches of philosophy: logic, humanism, existentialism, metaphysics, Epicureanism, materialism, stoicism, and many more. But according to Judeo-Christian tradition, the very foundation of wisdom is fixed upon the inerrant, divinely inspired Bible, making any school of thought founded upon another means destined for futility.[7] All of creation, including the heavens, the earth, and the world system now in place, is passing away, but God's words do not change with societal changes. Instead, they endure forever.[8]

Unveiling the Occult's Deception

The second counterfeit means our adversary uses to divert humans from God's truth is through the *occult*, a word derived from a Latin root meaning "hidden" and defined as "esoteric, supernatural beliefs and practices which reach beyond the scope of organized religion and science."[9]

In the Age of Enlightenment of the seventeenth century, occult practices such as alchemy, astrology, and magic came to be seen as antithetical to the burgeoning field of science. A revival of the occult sprang up in the nineteenth and early twentieth centuries with schools of thought such as Spiritualism and Theosophy, as people came to see that some experiences were not subject to scientific investigation or rational explanation. Examples of common occult practices at the time included necromancy through mediums at séances and through spirit boards as well as divination through interpreting the zodiac, tarot card readings, fortune-telling, and rune casting, to name a few. A second revival of occultism has sprung up in the late twentieth and early twenty-first centuries, with the New Age Movement and Wicca as prominent examples. Traditional Judeo-Christian beliefs forbid these practices, claiming that although sometimes occult practices yield legitimate information and power to their practitioners, their source is otherworldly spiritual agents of chaos with whom we are at war.[10] Essentially, occult practices are akin to acts of treason, in which traitors side with the enemy in order to curry their favor and gain knowledge, power, and influence through illegitimate means.

Balancing Science and Faith

The final common means the enemy uses to attack God's truth is scientific knowledge. The word *science* has evolved over time, originating from the Latin *scientia*, which simply meant "knowledge." Science today is generally conceptualized as collective attempts to provide explanations of phenomena in the natural world using facts that have been confirmed through observation and proper experimentation. But it is interesting to note that, historically, the only natural sciences that were part of standard university curriculum until the 1800s were geometry and astronomy.

In the 1800s, German universities employed the concept of *Wissenschaft*, which broadly redefined science as a legitimate area of study oriented toward a particular object and possessing appropriate methods of investigation. Hence, as in the time of the High Middle Ages, when theology was considered "the queen of the sciences," within this system of *Wissenschaft*, theology was once again considered a science with an object of study (God and his actions on earth) and a means for study (the Bible and general revelation).

While many today believe the natural sciences and theology to be at odds with each other, the two fields of study actually examine completely different aspects of reality. Whereas science concerns the natural world, theology is concerned with the supernatural world and its relationship to the natural world. By definition, the supernatural is above and beyond the natural, making it inaccessible to the same observations and testing employed by science to examine the natural world. Recognizing the value of scientific inquiry while maintaining a firm grasp on spiritual convictions allows for a balanced perspective that appreciates the contributions of both realms to human understanding and well-being. The integration model posits that scientific and religious knowledge can not only coexist but also complement each other, as scientific discoveries reveal the complexity and majesty of God's creation.[11]

A quote from the late British physician–turned–Christian pastor Martyn Lloyd-Jones serves as an appropriate transition from Step 10 to Step 11:

The only way to fight and to repel the enemy is to take up this Sword of the Spirit, which is the Word of God. If you are not certain that it is the Word of God, if you do not rely utterly, absolutely

*upon it, if you do not believe it is inerrant, then you have a bro-
ken sword in your hand, and you are already defeated by your
enemy. Take this sword and use it in the power of the Spirit, and
I care not what universities or scholars or anything else may arise
against you.*[12]

Step 11: Holy Scripture

*We read holy scripture regularly and asked God for the will and strength
to obey it.*

Committing to Sacred Truth

Having decided to seek knowledge and wisdom only from the
established teachings considered sacred by their chosen religious
faith, patients may now appropriate these teachings by making
a commitment to reading scripture regularly. Since deceit is the
number one tool used by spiritual enemies, the best means of
detecting deception is to have a firm grasp of the truth contained
within the full counsel of God. If patients are going to learn to
fight as soldiers in this spiritual war and ultimately win, they
must develop the discipline to train their minds with the ultimate
source of truth—holy scripture from the higher power they have
identified in their earnest search.

Admittedly, like all training, this is difficult, especially since the
world offers so many enticing substitutes with which a patient can
fill their time. It takes commitment and setting aside a regularly
scheduled time, knowing the costs of this investment will be offset
by the payment of larger dividends in future battles. Preferably, this
reading of scripture should be conducted daily, as it is metaphorically food for a patient's spirit, and like the physical food needed to
sustain their body, such nourishment is needed more than once or
twice a week for optimum spiritual health.[13]

Wielding the Sword of the Spirit

The Apostle Paul describes the final piece of armor available to patients from their higher power as the Sword of the Spirit. The other five pieces of armor Paul describes in Ephesians Chapter 6 are purely defensive in nature, but the sword is the one piece of battle gear at patients' disposal that acts as both a defensive and an offensive weapon. The sword is unique in its defensive nature: It is the one weapon that can hold back spiritual enemies themselves rather than just the strategic actions of their attack.

Paul uses the Greek term *machairan* here for sword, which refers to a short-bladed sword used by first-century Roman soldiers when in close contact with their enemies. In the same way, patients can use the Sword of the Spirit to fend off spiritual enemies who stealthily make their way up close to whisper lies in patients' ears and tempt them with the lust of the flesh, the lust of the eyes, and the pride of life.

Recall that the first piece of armor granted to patients by their higher power was the Belt of Truth, which was the foundational piece of soldiers' uniforms, signifying their acceptance of and commitment to the battle they faced. Hence, the aspect of truth the belt represents is also foundational in nature, namely that there is a God who is more powerful than patients and who is also willing to help them in their battles with illness and other tribulations in life. At this point, patients also embraced the truth that there are other malevolent spiritual beings who are at war with their higher power and that illness is one of the means these unseen enemies utilize to target mankind. But the aspect of truth represented by the Sword of the Spirit is that which is revealed by God in holy Scripture:[14]

For the Word of God is alive and powerful. It is sharper than the sharpest two-edged sword, cutting between soul and spirit, between joint and marrow. It exposes our innermost thoughts and desires.[15]

In the Bible, the phrase "the Word of God" is often employed to describe God's written words that the faithful believe were given to its writers by divine inspiration from God's Spirit. In the original Greek translation of the New Testament, there are two different terms that translate to "word." The first is *logos*, meaning the full, inerrant written counsel given under inspiration by God. The second is *rhema* (utterance), which refers to very specific portions of the written Word of God, and this is the term with which the Sword of the Spirit is concerned.

In close interpersonal battles with their unseen enemies, patients must use specific portions of scripture that are tailored to particular forms of spiritual attack. While there are a handful of useful techniques to resist the Devil, the one demonstrated by Jesus to make him flee is *rhema*, the sharp and agile Word of God.

Learning from Jesus's Example

At the beginning of his ministry, Jesus was an unknown thirty-year-old Jewish carpenter of humble origins from the backwater Galilean town of Nazareth. No one, including members of his own family, would have ever suspected that he would become someone great, someone whose teachings would affect the lives of billions of people for thousands of years. I surmise that Satan, while patrolling the earth, may have first suspected that Jesus was the redeemer sent by God after Jesus's baptism in the Jordan River, at which time the veil between the physical and spiritual realms was lifted temporarily, and God verbally proclaimed who Jesus was.[16] Immediately afterward, Jesus was compelled by God's Spirit to retreat into the harsh, barren wilderness of Judea for a forty-day period of testing, because this is the only means by which faith is proven genuine.[17] It is not a sin to be tempted—it is how one responds to the temptation that can be sinful. Scripture says that Jesus himself was "tempted in every way, just as we are—yet he did not sin."[18] Satan saw God's testing of Jesus for righteousness as an opportunity to turn temptation into sin, because Jesus was undoubtedly physically and emotionally exhausted, having endured in a rocky, dusty landscape without eating for forty days. But Jesus was not ignorant of the enemy's schemes, for he knew Satan to be a liar who prowls the earth looking for weak and weary prey.[19] When Satan got close to him, Jesus knew he had to wield the Sword of the Spirit to repel the enemy.

As recounted in the New Testament Gospels of Matthew and Luke, the Devil first enticed Jesus to use his God-given abilities to turn stones strewn on the barren Judean landscape into bread. Jesus responded by using a rhema sword—he quoted Scripture. Next, Satan asked Jesus to throw himself off the highest point of the Temple in Jerusalem so that God's angels could save him, proving to the throngs who had rejected him that he was indeed the Son of God. Jesus again responded by quoting Scripture. Finally, after unsuccessfully appealing to Jesus's unmet physical and emotional needs, Satan attempted to entice Jesus to fall victim to pride by offering him "all the kingdoms of the world and their glory" in exchange for his illegitimate worship of a false god, Satan himself. This final time, Jesus not only quoted Scripture but also commanded Satan to leave, after which, Scripture says, Satan "left [Jesus] until a more opportune time."[20]

The more patients utilize this same sword that Jesus used, the more they will be able to recognize subtle attacks by the enemy and then successfully fight their daily battles with invisible spiritual foes.

Transforming Through Renewal

Spiritual breakthrough occurs suddenly as patients first recognize the truth and surrender their lives and their will to that of their identified higher power. Transformation, on the other hand, comes gradually as patients live out the truth in their daily lives, renewing their minds regularly with the truths of scripture. This transformation involves a continuous process of growth and change in which patients align their thoughts and values with God's will.

The gradual process of *sanctification*, in which God transforms believers back to his original image-bearers, saves them from the power of sin. In prayer, Jesus modeled how to accomplish this by asking God to "Sanctify them by the truth; your Word is truth."[21] As tempting and alluring as it may be, patients must be vigilant not to conform to the behavior and customs of this world system; friendship with the world makes one an enemy of God.[22] Instead, as the Apostle Paul admonished believers, "Let God transform you into a new person by changing the way you think. Then you will learn to know God's will for you, which is good and pleasing and perfect."[23]

Transformation occurs from the inside out. First, it occurs mentally by the regular practice of patients renewing their minds with holy scripture, and then, eventually, it occurs on the outside when believers receive glorified, eternal bodies that the Bible says "will shine like the sun in the kingdom."[24] In fact, Scripture adds, "The sufferings of this present time are not worthy to be compared with the glory which shall be revealed in us."[25]

The importance of a renewed mind is not only that it thinks correctly but also that it values and treasures God's will, leading to a life that spontaneously reflects his purposes. A regenerate spirit and a continually renewed mind, washed and cleansed by daily reading of holy scripture, enable patients to subdue the sinful physical desires of "the flesh" and control their bodies. Just as a river will gradually cut away stone, regular reading of scripture cuts away the unnecessary and sinful parts of our physical nature, what the Bible calls the "spiritual circumcision."[26]

When I was a child, there was a public service ad campaign encouraging kids to eat healthfully by reminding them, "You are what you eat." As a physician, I have come to believe that that statement is largely true. As a doctor of the soul, I have also come to believe the much more profound truth that "you are what you think."[27] Science is finally catching up with what many people have known for centuries: Thoughts are things.

Neuroscientists have now proven that thoughts exist as electrical impulses and chemical reactions in the brain, and actually have mass. The sum total of patients' thoughts comprises their attitudes, which in turn lead to their actions, proving the old saying, "The thought is the father of the deed." This is why it is so vital for patients to learn to regulate their thoughts.

But renewing the mind goes beyond thinking; it also includes valuing what is good, acceptable, and perfect. This profound change in how patients assess and value things will lead to spontaneous godly behavior. The renewed mind helps patients discern the will of God, which includes both his sovereign will (everything that comes to pass) and his moral will (what he commands in Scripture that does not always come to pass due to humans exercising self-will). The goal of Step 11 is to align one's life with God's moral will through regular reading and then application of holy scripture. In developing this spiritual discipline, patients' spontaneous behavior in their daily lives should increasingly reflect a transformed mind that naturally aligns with God's will. It is ironic that when patients are utterly submitted, even enslaved, to the revealed will of God in scripture, they become radically free.[28] Patients are now liberated from conformity to duty-driven external standards of morality and finally free to love to do what they ought to do.

It doesn't matter where patients start in their reading of scripture, because as the Bible says, "all Scripture is inspired by God and is useful to teach us what is true and to make us realize what is wrong in our lives."[29] However, many people find it helpful to have a daily reading plan available from an app. There's no wrong way to do this spiritual exercise; the point is to start somewhere and then continue feasting on this spiritual food every day.[30]

Step 12: Prayer and Meditation

We sought to improve our conscious contact with God by practicing the daily discipline of scheduled and systematic prayer and meditation of all sorts.

Entering God's Presence

We have seen that God communicates to his human children by means of written scripture and the utter importance of tapping into this resource regularly. But there is a vital, final step, involving a two-way communication between patients and their higher power. Most call it *prayer*, which, incredible as it may seem, affords patients the awesome privilege of entering God's throne room and personally interacting with the loving King of the Universe.[31]

The ultimate litmus test of patients' progress in their spiritual journey is the character and quality of their prayer life. Just as patients will intentionally set aside time for people whom they love, they must likewise carve out time for God, who is invisible and will not clamor for their attention like their human relatives and friends. One approach many people utilize is having daily "quiet time" first thing in the morning, before the world is awake and the busy day begins with all its demands on our time. Jesus modeled placing a high priority on prayer to his heavenly Father and seemed to always carve out time to pray during his slightly more than three years of public ministry. In fact, he was in the habit of rising before dawn to pray each day.[32] He also withdrew from crowds often, to spend time alone in prayer, sometimes for an entire night.

Patients should realize that prayer is not some rote, magical incantation. It's important not to rely too heavily on memorized formal and ritualistic prayers, as they tend to be what Jesus called "meaningless repetitions" or "empty phrases."[33] Prayer is more about expression, communication, and relationship with the divine than it is the actual words uttered. The goal is not to know about God but rather to know God personally and intimately.

God has provided patients with spiritual armor to use against their spiritual enemies, but this armor is not maximally effective unless patients are at all times in fellowship with God, receiving strength, power, and protection from him. Jesus taught his followers that people "ought always to pray and not to faint [i.e., give up]."[34]

While there is no right way to pray, the Apostle Paul recommends that we all "pray in the Spirit on all occasions with all kinds of prayers."[35] Although perhaps it is ideal to maintain unfettered, constant contact with the divine, it is admittedly quite difficult in actual practice to pray without ceasing at all times in busy twenty-first-century society.[36] Still, a constant conversation with God is possible when he is given unrestricted access to your everyday life.

For example, circumstances that are joyous present an opportunity to express thankfulness to God. Other circumstances may thrust sickness, pain, and suffering upon patients, presenting opportunities for them to express their feelings to God and to ask for his ever-present help in times of trouble.[37] The main point the Apostle Paul is trying to make here is that patients are to be utterly dependent upon God moment by moment, because he is sovereign, omnipotent, and sustains all things.[38] Paul is also instructing his readers to employ every kind of prayer throughout their busy days: secret prayer, public prayer, church prayer, memorized formal professions of faith, common prayer, spontaneous prayer, and even prayers of groaning without any utterance or verbalization.

Crafting a Prayerful Discipline

While patients should pray moment by moment throughout the day, as the Spirit leads them, it is also wise to develop the spiritual discipline of daily prayer by having a scheduled and prioritized quiet time using a systematic approach, just as in the spiritual discipline of daily scripture reading. Patients must try different approaches and come up with the best system that works for them, but I will briefly describe one suggested template that many have found helpful over the years.

A useful first step for patients to begin their time of prayer is to humbly *confess their wrongs* to their higher power. This is vital, because patients are instructed to "come boldly to the throne of our gracious God," but only if they, themselves, are viewed as righteous before God through Jesus's sacrifice for them and regular confession of their sins.[39] While the Bible states that, at times, sickness is due to God's anger at patients' sin,[40] it also implies that refusing to confess sin contributes to sickness and suffering, or at least hinders resolution of these.[41] "But if we confess our sins," Scripture says, "he is faithful and righteous, forgiving us our sins and cleansing us from all unrighteousness."[42] Confession removes this greatest roadblock to patients' prayers and enables them to boldly approach God's throne of grace.

The next step in a prayerful quiet time is *praise*, in which patients adore God for his many wonderful attributes and character traits. Suggestions are to praise him for his goodness, patience, love, wisdom, greatness, knowledge, power, holiness, glory, and grace, among others. Praise naturally flows into the next step—*thanksgiving*.

When patients offer thanks to God for all that he has done for and given to them, they cultivate an attitude of gratitude. They recognize that God is the source from whom all blessings flow. Everything belongs to God, and everything patients possess has come from God as a gracious gift from a loving heavenly Father.[43] This step of giving thanks may naturally bring to mind things that are lacking in patients' lives. Hence, this stage flows into the next one, which is called *supplication.*

Sometimes erroneously called *petition*, supplication differs from that more formal and structured request to an authority in that it is more personal and emotional, expressing a spirit of humility and dependence upon God. This humble seeking of help, guidance, or blessings is not selfish. God is a loving Father, who actually wants patients to ask him for these things, and who also delights in granting them the desires of their heart when the desires are in concert with his will.[44] Scripture says, "In every circumstance and in everything, by prayer and supplication with thanksgiving, continue to make your wants known to God."[45]

Having prayed for their own needs and wants, patients should then turn to the needs of others who come to their mind or, preferably, who are on a prayer list patients keep as they encounter people suffering. This step is called *intercession*, and it is very important, because the people of God are likened to a body with parts that have different functions and varying degrees of honor but which are nevertheless interdependent upon each other for the body to function optimally.[46] This is one of the reasons that patients should be encouraged to seek out a like-minded community and not neglect meeting together.[47] Scriptures state that when people of a faith community confess their sins to each other and pray for each other, it facilitates the healing of the patients offering the prayers. In addition to this personal benefit, patients can also rest assured that, if they are walking in righteousness, their own earnest prayers for others will have great power and produce wonderful results.[48] The final reason for patients to intercede for others in daily prayer is the reality that we are all engaged in the same fight with our invisible spiritual foes.[49]

Listening in Stillness

So far, my description of patients' time of prayer has involved patients doing most of the talking. But, as stated earlier, one goal of prayer is to have fellowship with the divine, so there must also be time to wait and listen for a response from God. Investing a few moments in some deep, diaphragmatic breathing exercises can help patients quiet their minds and filter out any internal or external distractions in order to have a reverential focus on God alone, rest in him, and wait patiently for his response.[50]

Although waiting may seem like a boring and passive process, Scripture promises the rewards of strength and increased physical vitality for those who do so.[51] While training themselves in the discipline of listening, patients will come to realize that God's Spirit usually speaks in a "still, small voice," according to Scripture, so they must "not be hasty to speak" and instead let their words be few.[52] Patience is described as one of the evidences or "the fruit" of the Holy Spirit, and waiting and listening quietly in prayer helps develop this trait.

Meditating on Eternal Truths

Many spiritual practitioners over the years have found it helpful to end their quiet time of prayer by reading portions of holy scripture, as God clearly speaks through his written word. Often, reading through the Psalms proves particularly valuable because they display such a wide range of relatable human emotions. But reading scripture should not be seen as a task to be completed. Instead, it should be viewed as a slow-paced, methodical endeavor in which patients meditate upon the truths they encounter.

Unlike the still, quiet mind of the waiting stage, during this meditation, the mind is very active, pondering spiritual things. If patients meditate upon scripture regularly, it eventually becomes inscribed on what the Bible calls the "tablets of their hearts," where it can continually renew their minds and be used as a weapon against spiritual foes.[53]

Two Old Testament heroes of the Jewish faith, Joshua and King David, believed Scripture to be so important to the spiritual life that they both urged their readers to meditate upon it "day and night."[54] Contrary to New Age beliefs about the practice of meditation, true meditation for spiritual purposes does not involve emptying the mind but rather filling it with truths learned from the God of their understanding through prayer and reading scripture.

One final thought on prayer: Studies have shown that most healthcare professionals are not only hesitant to discuss spiritual matters with their patients but also reluctant to pray for patients openly. This is more likely due to healthcare providers being uncomfortable with the condition of their own spiritual life, because studies also show that most patients would welcome discussing such matters and praying with their providers.[55]

It is my strong belief that physicians and other healthcare providers are no different from their patients in that they, too, have a personal responsibility to develop their own spiritual beliefs and practices. In fact, I believe that clinicians have an even greater responsibility to do so if they genuinely desire to be of the utmost help to the patients whom they are called to serve. After all, if the blind lead the blind, both will fall into a ditch.[56] Conversely, spiritually mature clinicians should look for opportunities to model prayer with their patients, for their patients, and over their patients whenever clinically appropriate.

Prayer is indeed a spiritual duty, but it is so much more than that.

Scripture tells us that God "delights in the prayers of the upright [genuine followers]."[57] Ultimately, prayer is a wonderful privilege to fellowship with God; it is the ultimate expression of the spiritual life intent on healing, health, and true wholeness.

Epilogue

YOU WILL BE
COMPLETELY HEALED

In the prologue of this book, I asked you to imagine yourself coming to my medical office on referral for a treatment-resistant illness unresponsive to multiple standard-of-care treatments. You were given the diagnosis of a spiritual condition that was terminal but given hope for a cure by a famous yet controversial physician I happen to know. But before seeing him, I asked you to read this book. Okay, good—you read the book, and now it's finally time to see the physician who has the cure for your terminal illness. You make your way into the medical building, step onto the elevator, and press the button for the top floor. As the elevator doors open, you are in awe of the beauty of his office, which occupies the entire floor.

With a bit of trepidation, you walk toward an inviting, almost palatial, office with an open door, emanating a bright yet soothing light. You hesitate, until a friendly voice invites you to come inside and have a seat. "Hello there," says an unassuming man with a gentle and kind countenance. Not tall nor handsome, this man nevertheless exudes an aura of compassion, competence, and authority.

His eyes are intense, seeming to peer straight into your soul, but they are kind and nonjudgmental at the same time. You are drawn to him.

"I am Joshua Rapha. Dr. McCormack told me all about you. He told me you want to be healed. I'm so pleased you agreed to meet with me—not everyone he refers to me follows through with the referral. I am confident that what I have to offer will heal you."

Dr. Rapha then asks, "Are you willing to trust my diagnosis of your malady and also to comply with my instructions for your healing, however unconventional, uncomfortable, or seemingly unreasonable? I must warn you that procuring this breakthrough cure goes against the grain of standard medical practice and can have grave consequences. You must be fully informed of the risks before consenting. You risk getting fired from your job, losing relationships, becoming an object of ridicule or scorn, getting canceled, having your freedoms taken away, or even losing your life in the process. But the benefit of being snatched from death, having new life, and a life even more abundant than before, far outweighs these risks."

After momentarily counting the costs, you consent to the cure. His warnings certainly seem hyperbolic to you, but what choice do you have when your very life hangs in the balance?

"Excellent," Dr. Rapha responds with a warm smile. "First, come to me with your ears wide open. Listen, and you will find life.[1] Now look at that mosaic on the wall," he says as he motions to a tiled mosaic bearing a pole with a bronze snake intertwined in it. You think it strange, but you comply with his request, nevertheless. With an air of great authority, he pronounces, "I hereby promise that if you look upon this serpent and believe you will be healed, it shall be done unto you!"

You instantaneously feel a sense of peace you have never experienced. You are altogether surprised and think your mind is playing tricks on you. *Who is this guy?* you wonder. He seems like a benevolent mix of P. T. Barnum and Franz Mesmer. The experience is over, and you are escorted back to the elevator, which returns to the first floor, where my office is located.

Upon reentering my office, I perform some additional tests and confirm that you are indeed healed of your terminal illness. Congratulations are in order. You, however, are understandably confused by what just transpired, stating, "I don't get it. All I did was look at the caduceus on his wall. That makes no logical sense!"

"Please sit down," I say, gesturing to a chair in my private office. I explain that it was not a caduceus you looked upon in Dr. Rapha's office. The caduceus is a short staff entwined by two serpents surmounted by wings, which was a symbol of commerce carried by Hermes in Greek mythology. Nor was it the rod of Asclepius, the symbol of modern medicine derived from the ancient Greek cult of the god of healing, who carried a snake-entwined staff.

"Then what in the world was it that I looked at in his office?" you frustratingly inquire.

I explain that, nearly 3,500 years ago, when Moses led the Israelites out of Egypt into the Sinai wilderness on the way to the Promised Land, the people soon became disheartened, and in their lack of faith, they grumbled against Moses. They failed to realize that their own sins were the reason for their difficulties, instead choosing to point the finger at Moses. As a consequence of their disobedience, God sent venomous snakes into the camp as a form of judgment, and many began to perish. This calamity made it clear to the people that they were the ones at fault, prompting them to approach Moses, admit their wrongdoing, and plead for God's mercy.

When Moses interceded on their behalf, God directed him to craft a bronze serpent, fasten it to a pole, and raise it up so that the people could be healed by looking at it.[2] Through this, God was imparting a lesson about faith. Logically, it made no sense that gazing at a bronze figure could cure someone of a deadly snakebite, yet that was precisely what God commanded. Healing required an act of faith in God's plan, and the serpent on the pole served as a symbol of their sin, which had led to their suffering.

Jesus indicated that this bronze serpent was a foreshadowing of him: "And as Moses lifted up the bronze snake on a pole in the wilderness, so the Son of Man must be lifted up, so that everyone who believes in him will have eternal life."[3] The serpent, a symbol of sin and judgment, was lifted up from the earth and put on a tree, which was a symbol of a curse.[4] The lifted-up and cursed serpent symbolized Jesus, who takes away sin from everyone who looks to him in faith, just as the Israelites had to look to the upraised symbol in the wilderness. Jesus voluntarily became a curse for us, even though he was blameless and sinless—the one whom the Scripture calls the spotless Lamb of God. "God made him who had no sin to be sin for us, so that in him we might become the righteousness of God."[5] Mankind should exercise faith by looking to Jesus lifted up on a Roman cross in order to be saved from death, the wages of our collective sins.

Similarly, it took an act of faith for a first-century paralytic man, who for thirty-eight years had tried both the traditional and even superstitious and unconventional approaches to healing, to be made whole by Jesus. Jesus met this desperate man at a pool he came to live adjacent to because he believed the water could cure him when it was supposedly stirred by an angel.[6] The paralytic's initial faith in medicine and a supposedly miraculous body of water was misguided, however. This account underscores the importance of stepping out and relying upon faith when traditional modes of healing have proven unsuccessful. But it also underscores the importance of where one's faith is directed. After all, when it comes to our physical, emotional, social, and spiritual health, we all put our faith in something. It does not mean that patients should not seek out the help of physicians and their arts of medicine and surgery when appropriate. Instead, it means we should recognize where the only offer of complete healing comes from—God, the Great Physician, who is sovereign over all things, including our health.

I then inquire, "Did Dr. Rapha ask you to do anything else besides gaze at the serpent on the staff?"

You ponder the question momentarily and then respond, "Yeah, he asked me to believe that I could be healed."

I go on to explain that, although unconventional, Dr. Rapha believed that there was a spiritual component to your sickness that had not been addressed, so he was performing a test to assess your degree of faith. It was your faith, albeit small, that blew open the door, allowing healing to rush in.

I pause to let you soak it all in. You sit speechless for a few moments and then question, "Dr. McCormack, who exactly is this Dr. Rapha, and how did just looking at the image of the bronze snake on a pole lead to my healing?"

I go on to explain that Dr. Rapha is in fact *the* Great Physician, the Savior of mankind himself, who appeared to you in human form to veil his glory, which no human can witness and live. "I understand that it is difficult to fathom," I say. "From here, it is now your personal responsibility to earnestly search and decide who this God is."

"Don't get me wrong—I am incredibly grateful he cured my fatal disease, but why am I still in pain?" you ask. "Couldn't he have taken that away, too?"

I sigh as I struggle for words to succinctly explain the answer to your difficult question. "The reason for your continued pain is that according to the Christian religion, the war between God and rebellious created spirit beings rages on, despite the fact that Jesus Christ came to reclaim his land 2,000 years ago, disarming our spiritual foes and making a public spectacle of them. The ultimate outcome of the war has already been determined—God wins.

"Nevertheless, Christianity, Judaism, and Islam all also concede that although the verdict has been pronounced against the bad guys, since they have yet to be sentenced, they continue to sow chaos and promote sin, sickness, and death until the day God returns in final judgment. As a psychiatrist, it is my professional opinion that these spiritual malefactors are delusional and actually think they can win."

I go on to explain that none of us is immune. Suffering is an inevitable part of human life according to Jesus, but he also provides solid assurance of victory through him.[7] Jesus's assurance that he has "overcome the world" reminds us that God remains in control, even when life feels chaotic or unbearable. His disciples, though soon to face profound grief over his crucifixion, were reminded that their sorrow on Friday and Saturday would turn to joy at Jesus's resurrection on Sunday.[8] Followers of Jesus today will likewise experience moments of grief, sorrow, pain, and suffering in their brief lives that are "light" and "momentary" in comparison to the eternal glory awaiting them.[9] Jesus compares our suffering to childbirth: Though painful, it produces indescribable and lasting joy once the child is born, analogous to the joy believers will experience when Jesus returns to occupy his world and glorify believers.[10] By focusing on the "unseen"—the eternal life and hope promised through Christ—believers can find strength to endure trials. This perspective allows suffering to become a transformative process, shaping faith and character while directing attention to the eternal rewards.[11]

Knowing these truths, you can reframe your pain and suffering not as a sign of God's absence but as an opportunity to trust him more deeply, grow spiritually, and develop the fortitude needed to endure with faith and hope. The prophet Isaiah stated that even though God gives you adversity and suffering, "he will still be with you to teach you." In fact, even in the darkest valleys of life, he will never leave you. One day your suffering will end forever, and you will see your teacher with your own eyes and hear him with your own ears.[12] Until then, you can learn to exercise faith and even say to God, "My suffering was good for me, for it taught me to pay attention to your decrees."[13] Anything, even suffering and seemingly adverse circumstances, can be a good thing in the context of eternity, if God is at work in it.

Patients who have accepted the reality of suffering in their own life and the world in general and who have earnestly sought a higher power to help are on the right track to healing. But there are additional steps to healing that many are either unaware of or unwilling to take. For those patients who have surrendered their will and life to their higher power, performed a demolition of demonic strongholds in their spiritual house, and taken steps to draw closer to God, an offer of greater healing is free and readily available. In particular, those who have placed their faith in Jesus Christ's death on the cross as payment for their own sins are rescued from the penalty of sin and death, which they deserve for breaking God's laws. But their healing is not yet complete. Physical and emotional pain, sicknesses, and, ultimately, physical death remain realities.

So, what is the reason we continue to experience suffering, despite having a growing spiritual life and the testimony of Scripture that God's kingdom has come to earth already? The theological principle of "already but not yet" refers to the idea that although certain aspects of God's promises and kingdom are already in place, we do "not yet" see the kingdom in its full glory.[14] In this paradigm, it is believed that the kingdom of God was inaugurated through the first coming of Jesus Christ, resulting in the forgiveness of sins, a new relationship with God, and the Holy Spirit being sent to indwell believers after Jesus ascended. Despite these present realities, the ultimate fulfillment of God's kingdom is still in the future, including the complete eradication of sin, suffering, and death.

Grasping the "already but not yet" aspect of reality will help you navigate the tension between current ongoing suffering and future hope of the complete fulfillment of God's kingdom. This perspective can foster resilience and hope amid the trials and suffering you experience on your spiritual journey through this life.

Scripture backs up this view that despite certainty of the outcome of this cosmic war, "we do not yet see all things put" in subjection "under him."[15] Christians, Jews, and Muslims alike look forward in faith to that promised day when God enacts his final judgment, rightly puts all things in subjection under his anointed King, and ends sin, sickness, death, and all warfare forever.

While Jesus walked on the earth, he did not fear sickness or death and neither should we, because they are inevitable realities we all will face. But Jesus knew sickness and death were consequences of sin and that his own voluntary sacrificial death and subsequent resurrection would inaugurate their defeat. This is why, for example, Jesus did not shy away from approaching and laying his hands on those with very contagious diseases, such as leprosy. In another instance, when he was told his good friend Lazarus had a serious illness, Jesus chose to stay where he was for two additional days, during which time Lazarus died. Then Jesus decided to go to Bethany to visit Lazarus's sisters, Mary and Martha, even though only days prior the people in that region had tried to kill him.

"Martha met Jesus as he was approaching their home, and she rebuked him: 'Lord, if only you had been here, my brother would not have died.'"[16]

When Jesus responded that Lazarus would rise again, Martha believed her brother would "rise when everyone else rises, at the last day." Jesus knew he was moments away from raising Lazarus from the dead, yet he wept with Mary, Martha, and the rest of the mourners because he both had compassion on them and was angry at the sin and death that so negatively impacted those who loved Lazarus. Jesus proved he was indeed the great high priest who is able "to empathize with our weaknesses."[17] Jesus then displayed his authority and power over death by performing his greatest miracle, raising Lazarus from the dead after four days.

I explain to you it is important to note that Jesus did not rush over to Bethany to heal Lazarus the moment he learned the man was sick. Jesus did eventually perform the healing of Lazarus, just later than they all had hoped and expected. "God will do the same for you," I continue, "but you may have to wait and endure suffering as he works all things together for the ultimate good of all whom he loves."

I point out that while God certainly can, and sometimes does, heal patients' physical and mental illnesses while they are on earth, often he does not. Nevertheless, he still cares deeply and comforts those who are suffering. Most importantly, he promises that one day he will provide complete healing when believers receive their eternal glorified bodies that will be impervious to sin, sickness, and death.

We confidently and joyfully look forward to sharing God's glory. We can rejoice, too, when we run into problems and trials, for we know that they help us develop endurance. And endurance develops strength of character, and character strengthens our confident hope of salvation. And this hope will not lead to disappointment. For we know how dearly God loves us, because he has given us the Holy Spirit to fill our hearts with his love. When we were utterly helpless, Christ came at just the right time and died for us sinners.[18]

Still clearly grappling with the profundity of the experience, you exclaim, "I can't believe that all it took for me to be saved from death was to look at that symbol on his wall and believe—it seems so easy."

I wrap up our session with encouraging words: "For today, just be incredibly thankful for the gift of healing and the new lease on life. This new life is a walk, not a sprint, and you are just starting your way on the long, narrow road. More will be revealed along the way, so just be patient for now. I am so very pleased you have bravely chosen this path, and you are now ready to move forward in your journey to wholeness, despite the known risks."

Closing Reflections

As we reach the end of this journey together, I hope you feel a spark of something new—a stirring of hope, a whisper of possibility. Through these pages, we've explored the unseen forces that shape our lives, the spiritual battles that rage beyond our perception, and the profound healing that awaits those who dare to seek it. You've walked with me through the shadows of doubt and skepticism, past the chaos of a world at war with itself, and into the light of a truth that promises wholeness.

This book began with a question: Do you want to be healed? Perhaps, like the patient in my prologue, your initial answer was a hesitant nod, unsure of what that healing might entail. Now, having ventured through the realities of spiritual warfare and the transformative power of faith, I invite you to consider that question anew.

Healing—true, complete healing—is not just a distant dream. It's a promise, extended to you by the Great Physician himself.

But let's be clear: This journey doesn't end with the turn of the final page. It's just beginning. The path to wholeness is narrow, often steep, and rarely easy. It demands courage—to decide who you believe to be the highest spiritual power and at least examine the claims of the God who professes to be the omnipotent self-existent healer. After intensively studying medicine, history, theology, and psychology for many years, I have come to the conclusion that only one system of beliefs in the entire history of the world compellingly promises complete healing for all four aspects of the biopsychosocial-spiritual model of disease.

The result of my own earnest and thorough spiritual search has led this former worldly agnostic to now confidently and unashamedly follow Jesus of Nazareth, a Jew from the Roman province of Galilee who 2,000 years ago began a teaching and healing ministry in what is now modern-day Israel. This Jesus has become the most famous man in all of world history, with billions of followers believing his claims to be the Son of God and the long-awaited prophesied Messiah of God's chosen people, the Israelites. As C. S. Lewis so powerfully argued, Jesus is either Lord, lunatic, or liar. Jesus's thoroughly chronicled life and words leave no other possible conclusions. I urge you to examine the evidence—his life, his many well-documented miracles, his words, the prophecies fulfilled, the billions transformed—and choose for yourself. Your decision will echo beyond this moment, shaping your life and your eternity.

Since "God has given us this task of reconciling people to him,"[19] my heartfelt desire is that *Hidden Medicine* has ignited something within you—a hunger for spiritual truth, a resolve to live out the principles of Ruachiatry, and a passion to carry this hope to others.

By working through the 12 Steps of Ruachiatry, you can begin healing your accumulated spiritual wounds and then launch forward on a new path in submission to your higher power now acting as your ally. Periodically working through the steps, perhaps with a certified Ruachiatry coach or with patient-run meetings—similar to those of A.A. and N.A.—may provide extra support for those who desire it.

With newfound insight into the cosmic battle in which you are embroiled, realize that you're not meant to walk this path alone. Throughout my years as a psychiatrist, I've seen the power of community lift the broken and steady the weary. We are all fighting a common enemy, and we are all subject to the same problems of sickness, suffering, and eventual death. So, be careful not to view your problems in a personal and subjective manner, erroneously labeling them *my* problems, *my* sickness, *my* suffering, etc. Now that you're able to see things from the larger perspective of a cosmic war, you will be better able to take your focus off your personal suffering and recognize the great privilege of being allowed to take part in this Crusade of God against the spiritual forces of evil.

Choose a religious faith, regularly attend corporate worship services, and seek out fellow travelers—believers who can pray with you, challenge you, and stand with you against the enemy's schemes. Finally, resolve to stand firm as a warrior in the army of God and to also help your fellow soldiers to stand, because failure of any one of the soldiers in our unit is bound to negatively affect the entire campaign. After all, we soldiers of God are a mutually interdependent band of brothers and sisters who are stronger together than the forces that seek to tear us down. We're all soldiers in this cosmic battle, wounded yet called to fight, not just for ourselves but for those still lost in the fray. Your story, your healing, can become a beacon for the sick, the suffering, and the searching.

Healing, though, is a process—a sacred unfolding. You may still feel the sting of pain, the weight of suffering. That's the tension of the "already but not yet"—God's kingdom has broken into our world through Jesus, yet its fullness awaits his return. Today, your wounds may linger, but they are not the end of your story. In fact, no matter what your story has been to this point, the Great Physician stands ready to meet you where you are, to heal you, to lead you into a life more abundant than you've dared to imagine.

So, as you close this book, know this: You are not alone, and you are not without hope. Take that first step of faith—then the next one and so forth—drawing closer to the loving and all-powerful Highest Power. If you do so, this promise is certain: In his perfect timing and by his boundless grace, one day you will be completely healed.

ACKNOWLEDGMENTS

Writing *Hidden Medicine* has been a journey that revealed the profound impact that countless individuals have had on my life and work. This book would not exist without the wisdom, support, and inspiration of many, and it is with deep gratitude that I acknowledge their contributions.

First and foremost, to my family: Words cannot express the depth of my appreciation. Thank you for your understanding during the long hours I spent writing at night after work and on weekends. To my wife, Michelle: I appreciate your love and patience during this project. It has been a blessing to witness your own ongoing spiritual journey. To my children, Mary Caroline, Thomas, and Catherine: I have no greater joy than to see my children walking in the truth. I am so proud of each of you and am excited to see how God will guide each of your lives. Your love and faith amid our own family's spiritual battles inspire me. May this book remind you that walking closely with God brings refinement, strength, and victory through life's most difficult trials.

Thank you to the best and most supportive parents, Wayne and Eleanor. Your sacrifices gave Rob, Cathy, and me an education, experiences, a godly example, and opportunities that set us all up for success. I love you, Mom. I miss you, Dad.

My brother Rob and my friends Bob Beith and Todd McNeal have been steadfast supporters of this endeavor, and I am most grateful for having three godly men I call friends who stand in the gap with me, challenge me, and teach me.

My pastors, spiritual mentors, and churches have nurtured my faith and deepened my understanding of the unseen forces at work in our lives. To Pastor Stewart Simms, DMin, who baptized me and shepherded me as a young man starting my journey of faith. To Pastor David Mills, PhD, who first suggested I write this book and who, through his godly leadership and personal example of how to respond to intense spiritual warfare, inspired me and gave me a yearning to fulfill God's Great Commission. To my current pastor Dr. Josh Smith, who encouraged me, gave feedback, and shared his own publishing journey with me. I greatly treasure you three shepherds who God sent into my life. Your prayers and encouragement have been a source of strength throughout this journey.

My professional mentors and colleagues have profoundly shaped my understanding of medicine and psychiatry. To the faculty at Emory University and Duke University, where I received my medical education and training: Thank you for instilling in me the rigor and curiosity that have guided my career. To my handful of colleagues in medical school, particularly Dr. Eric Graham and Dr. Chris Kersey, who, early in my spiritual journey, would stay up with me late into the night having discussions about religion and spirituality. Special thanks to Dr. Charles Keith, professor emeritus of psychiatry at Duke, whose guidance during my residency opened my eyes to the complexities of the human mind and spirit.

I must also acknowledge the many patients I have had the privilege to serve over the years. Though your names are not mentioned, your journeys are woven into the fabric of these pages, and I am profoundly appreciative of the trust you placed in me. Special thanks to my nurse practitioner, Meredith Jones, who helped coordinate our clinical studies and holistically treat patients in our practice as the world's first Ruachiatry coach.

I would also like to thank Brent Cole, who gave invaluable guidance to this first-time author, edited the first manuscript, and introduced me to Justin Branch at Greenleaf Book Group. Thank you to my fantastic team at Greenleaf, especially my lead editor, Emma Watson; my substantive editor, Katherine Tomlinson; and my copy editor, Hayden Seder. Special thanks are due to Hannah Marlow for her patience in dealing with my many cover design revisions.

Finally, to you, the reader: Thank you for embarking on this journey with me. It is my hope that *Hidden Medicine* will not only inform but also inspire you to explore the hidden truths that can lead to true healing. May you find in these pages the courage to seek, the wisdom to discern, and the faith to trust in the Great Physician, who promises wholeness.

With heartfelt gratitude,
—Dr. Thomas W. McCormack, Jr.

NOTES

Prologue

1. 2 Corinthians 4:4.
2. John 8:44.
3. Psalm 146:8; Matthew 9:27–31; Mark 10:46–52; Mark 8:22–26; John 9:1–41.
4. Genesis 3:19; Ecclesiastes 12:7; Romans 6:23; Hebrews 9:27.
5. 2 Corinthians 8:9; 2 Peter 3:9.
6. John 5:2–9.
7. Ephesians 6:12.

Chapter 1

1. Quran 55:15.
2. George Engel, "The Need for a New Medical Model: A Challenge for Biomedicine," *Science* 196, no. 4286 (1977), 129–36, https://doi.org/10.1126/science.847460.
3. Perhaps it is not insignificant that the most respected historians—atheists, agnostics, and Christians alike—have repeatedly cited Jesus as the most significant figure in human history.
4. Luke 13:10–16.
5. Mark 9:17–27.
6. Luke 9:37–42.
7. Matthew 9:32–33.
8. Mark 5:1–20; Luke 8:26–39.
9. Including Christianity (31.2%), Islam (24.1%), Hinduism (15%), and Buddhism (6.9%).
10. Plato's Apology, 38a5–6.

Chapter 2

1. Genesis 3:15; Ephesians 6:12; 1 Timothy 4:7; 1 Timothy 6:12; 2 Corinthians 10:4; 2 Timothy 2:4.

2. Isaiah 14:13–14; Ezekiel 28:17.

3. John 10:10.

4. 2 Timothy 2:3; 1 Corinthians 9:24.

5. Ezekiel 28:14–15.

6. Exodus 20:3.

7. This is one among a number of reasons that I firmly believe we as a society should be very cautious about legalizing mind- and perception-altering substances for use by the general public without extensive research and medical oversight.

8. This quote is commonly attributed to Miguel de Cervantes, though it does not appear in his works verbatim. The phrase is derived from the Latin proverb *praemonitus, praemunitus*, and Cervantes's *Don Quixote* contains similar themes of preparation and wisdom.

Chapter 3

1. 1 Kings 19:12–13.

2. Acts 9:3–9.

3. James 4:6 (NIV); Proverbs 3:34.

4. Mark 10:23 (NLT).

5. 1 Corinthians 15:45.

6. Francis Thompson, "The Hound of Heaven," Project Gutenberg, https://www.gutenberg.org/files/30730/30730-h/30730-h.htm.

Chapter 4

1. Isaiah 46:10 (AMP).

2. John 16:33.

3. Jeremiah 29:11; Romans 8:28.

4. Surah Al A'raf 7:12; Surah Sad 38:76; Surah Al-Isra 17:61.

5. Matthew 13:35; 1 Peter 1:20.

6. Genesis 3:15 (NLT).

7. Ecclesiastes 33:11 (NLT).

8. C. S. Lewis, *Mere Christianity* (Scribner Paper Fiction, 1952).

9. Romans 8:21 (NLT).

10. Charles Baudelaire, "Le Joueur Généreux" (The Generous Gambler) from his 1864 collection *Petits Poèmes en Prose*.

11. Later Jewish writings, such as an Aramaic paraphrase of the Hebrew Bible called the Targum Pseudo-Jonathan, and Islamic traditions and commentators like Al-Tabari, describe Nimrod as a rebellious, powerful king who claimed divine status.

12. Flavius Josephus. *Antiquities of the Jews*, book 1, chapter 4, paragraph 2.

13. Genesis 10:10.

14. Genesis 11:4 (NLT).

15. Deuteronomy 32:8–9.

16. Genesis 12:3.

17. Genesis 16:1–16; 21:1–19.

18. Genesis 25:29–34; 27:1–36; 33:1–15.

19. Genesis 32:27–28.

20. Exodus 1:22; 2:1–10.

21. Numbers 13–36.

22. 1 Samuel 8.

23. Matthew 2:1–18.

24. Matthew 16:23.

25. *The Devil's Advocate*, directed by Taylor Hackford (Warner Bros. Pictures, 1997).

26. 2 Timothy 3:3–4 (NLT).

27. Psalm 139:16.

Chapter 5

1. C. S. Lewis, *Surprised by Joy: The Shape of My Early Life* (Harcourt Brace, 1955), 207.

2. 1 Samuel 5:2.

3. 1 Samuel 5:4.

4. 1 Samuel 5:4.

5. Although Zoroastrianism worships Ahura Mazda as its one true god, the religion is technically dualistic, with the world seen as a cosmic struggle between the supreme Ahura Mazda and the evil Angra Mainyu.

6. Matthew 12:43–45 (NKJV).

7. Daniel 10:6 (NLT).

8. Daniel 10:12–13 (NLT).

9. Daniel 10:20 (NLT).

10.   2 Kings 6:16.

11.   Billy Graham, *Angels* (Thomas Nelson Inc, 1995), 7–8.

12.   Isaiah 14:16–17 (NKJV).

13.   Luke 8:17 (NLT).

Chapter 6

1.   While this quote is widely attributed to Saint Augustine, there is no definitive evidence in his extant writings. The sentiment does align with his theology, particularly his reflections on the struggle with sin and the nature of human weakness, as seen in *Confessions*.

2.   Walt Kelly, *Pogo*, Earth Day poster, 1970.

3.   Romans 3:11–12 (ESV).

4.   1 Thessalonians 5:23.

5.   Genesis 2:7.

6.   Matthew 16:26; Luke 9:25.

7.   John 4:24; Romans 1:9.

8.   Genesis 1:27; John 4:24.

9.   Ephesians 2:1–5.

10.   Genesis 3:17–19.

11.   Isaiah 24:5–6; Romans 8:20–21.

12.   2 Peter 3:7; Matthew 24:35; Isaiah 65:17; Revelation 21:1.

13.   1 Corinthians 2:14 (AMP).

14.   Matthew 13:18.

15.   Ephesians 6:12 (TLB).

16.   1 Corinthians 1:18.

17.   Colossians 1:21.

18.   John 3:19.

19.   Genesis 3:4 (LEB).

20.   James 4:4.

21.   Romans 8:31.

22.   Ezekiel 34:11; Luke 19:10.

23.   Romans 6:2.

24.   Wilhelm Gensenius, *A Hebrew and English Lexicon of the Old Testament*, trans. Edward Robinson (Crocker and Brewster, 1836), 446.

25.   Colossians 1:13; Ephesians 6:10–18.

26.   2 Corinthians 3:18.

27.   Romans 12:2; Philippians 2:13.

28. Galatians 5:22–23.

29. Matthew 4:4 (CSB).

30. Isaiah 55:9; Revelation 21:4–5.

31. Titus 2:11–13.

32. Matthew 26:41.

33. Ephesians 6:16; James 1:14–15.

34. Galatians 5:16–17.

35. Romans 8:13.

36. Romans 12:1.

37. Romans 13:14.

38. Ephesians 4:22–31.

39. Lewis, *Mere Christianity*.

40. 1 John 2:15 (NIV).

41. Genesis 1:4, 10, 12, 18, 21, 25, 31.

42. Genesis 3:1–7.

43. 2 Corinthians 4:4; 1 John 5:19.

44. 1 John 2:16.

45. Job 1:7.

46. My gratitude to the late preacher Dr. Adrian Rogers for this reference.

47. 1 Kings 22:17; Ezekiel 34:5; Zechariah 10:2; Matthew 9:36; Mark 6:34.

48. This inscription is on a house in Hamelin, Germany, known as Rattenfangerhaus, which in English translates to "Rat Catcher's House" otherwise known as the Pied Piper's House.

49. 1 Peter 2:11.

50. Ephesians 2:19.

51. Ephesians 2:1–6.

52. John 16:33 (NKJV).

53. Romans 12:2; 1 John 2:15.

54. John 15:18–25; John 7:7.

55. 1 John 4:4 (NKJV).

56. Ephesians 6:16 (ESV); 1 John 2:16 (NIV).

57. Matthew 13:38; John 8:44; 1 John 3:10; Acts 13:10.

58. Ephesians 2:2; Ephesians 5:5; Colossians 3:6.

59. Proverbs 3:11–12; Hebrews 12:6–11.

60. Job 1:7; Job 2:2.

61. Luke 4:1–15; Matthew 4:1–11.

62. Genesis 25:29–34; Hebrews 12:15–17.

63. Romans 12:17–21; 1 Thessalonians 5:15; 1 Peter 3:9.

64. Ephesians 6:12 (NLT).

Chapter 7

1. Isaiah 29:16.

2. Isaiah 14:14.

3. 2 Peter 3:9.

4. Michael Heiser, *The Unseen Realm: Recovering the Supernatural Worldview of the Bible* (Lexham Press, 2015), 56–58.

5. Ezekiel 28:14–17.

6. Job 38:7.

7. Isaiah 14:13–14 (NLT).

8. 2 Corinthians 4:4.

9. 1 Peter 5:8; Ephesians 6:12.

10. Job 1–2.

11. Zechariah 3.

12. Revelation 12:10.

13. 1 John 2:1; Romans 8:34.

14. Romans 8:1 (NLT).

15. Genesis 3:15; Colossians 3:6.

16. Ephesians 4:31 (NKJV).

17. Matthew 5:22 (NLT); 1 John 3:15.

18. John 8:44.

19. 1 John 3:12.

20. Leonard Ravenhill, *Why Revival Tarries* (Bethany House Publishers, 1959).

21. John 8:44.

22. 2 Corinthians 11:14.

23. John 14:6.

24. Revelation 12:9 (EHV).

25. John 10:10 (NLT).

26. Genesis 32:28.

27. Genesis 3:1–5; Heiser, *The Unseen Realm*, 74–76.

28. 2 Corinthians 11:14.

29. John 8:34; Romans 6:16.

30. Genesis 3:1–6.

31. Matthew 4:1–11; Mark 1:12–13; Luke 4:1–13.

32. 1 Thessalonians 3:5.

33. 1 Corinthians 10:13.

34. James 1:3.

35. 1 Corinthians 15:47.

36. James 1:13.

37. Romans 8:17–18 (NLT).

38. 1 Corinthians 10:13; Philippians 4:7.

39. Ephesians 6:16.

40. Exodus 16:4; 2 Chronicles 32:31; John MacArthur, *The MacArthur New Testament Commentary: James* (Moody Publishers, 1998), 29–32.

41. 2 Corinthians 12:7.

42. Exodus 2:11–25.

43. Philippians 1:23–24.

44. Genesis 22:1–12.

45. 2 Corinthians 1:3–5.

46. John MacArthur, "The Purpose of Trials," Grace to You, June 8, 1986, https://www.gty.org/library/sermons-library/59-5/the-purpose-of-trials.

47. Alexander Maclaren, "Faith Tested and Crowned," Asermon.com, http://www.asermon.com/books/maclaren-fatih-tested-crowned.html.

48. Matthew 20:26–28.

49. Isaiah 14:13–14.

50. Luke 22:42; Matthew 26:39–43.

51. 2 Corinthians 4:4.

52. Ephesians 2:2.

53. Michael Heiser, *Demons: What the Bible Really Says About the Powers of Darkness* (Lexham Press, 2020), 168.

54. Luke 4:5–7; Matthew 4:8–10.

55. John 12:31; 14:30; 16:11.

56. Karl Marx and Frederick Engels, *Marx/Engels Collected Works*, vol. 1, trans. Clemens Dutt (International Publishers, 1975), 683–85.

57. 1 Peter 5:8.

58. Revelation 9:11.

59. Thomas Aquinas, *Summa Theologica*, First Part (Prima Pars), trans. Fathers of the English Dominican Province (Benziger Bros., 1947; reprint Christian Classics, 1981).

60. Heiser, *Demons*, 47–49.

61. Chad Bird, "The Devil in the Details of the Old Testament: Is Satan in the

Hebrew Bible?" 1517, January 18, 2022, https://www.1517.org/articles/the-devil-in-the-details-of-the-old-testament-is-satan-in-the-hebrew-bible.

62. Wisdom of Solomon 2:24 (RSV).

63. *The Life of Adam and Eve*, Biblical.ie, https://www.biblical.ie/page.php?fl=Apocrypha%2FLife_of_Adam_and_Eve.

64. Revelation 12:9 (NIV).

65. 1 John 4:4.

66. Matthew 25:41.

67. Matthew 13:42, among other verses.

68. Romans 3:23.

69. Romans 6:23.

70. Romans 5:12.

71. 2 Peter 3:9.

72. Ezekiel 28:16 (NKJV).

73. Luke 10:18 (NKJV).

74. Mark 9:48; Isaiah 66:24 (NLT).

Chapter 8

1. Matthew 25:41; Revelation 12:7.

2. C. S. Lewis, *The Screwtape Letters* (Barbour and Company, 1990), 9.

3. 1 Samuel 16:14–23.

4. Deuteronomy 32:17; Leviticus 17:7; Psalm 106:37.

5. Isaiah 40:22.

6. Job 38:4–7.

7. Hebrews 1:14.

8. Genesis 3:8.

9. Genesis 6:4 (NLT).

10. 2 Peter 2:4; Jude 1:6.

11. 1 Enoch 15:8–12.

12. Heiser, *Demons*, 168.

13. 1 John 3:8.

14. Genesis 11:1–9.

15. Psalm 82:1–8.

16. Isaiah 49:6.

17. Colossians 1:16.

18. Heiser, *Demons*, 133.

19. Colossians 2:15.

20. 2 Corinthians 1:22; 5:5; 1 Corinthians 6:19.

21. Matthew 9:32–33; 12:22; 17:15–18.

22. Mark 5:1–20; Luke 8:26–39; Acts 16:16–18.

23. 2 Corinthians 2:10–11; 2 Corinthians 11:3–4; 13–15; 1 Timothy 4:1–5; 1 John 4:1–3.

24. Luke 8:26–39 (NLT); Mark 5:1–20; Matthew 8:22–34.

25. Luke 8:31 (NLT).

26. Luke 8:35 (NLT).

27. Luke 8:39 (NLT).

28. For further study on this subject, I recommend the book *Demonic Foes*, authored by fellow psychiatrist Dr. Richard Gallagher. I agree with Dr. Gallagher's assertion that, while the modern scientific perspective often interprets demonic possession as psychological or neurological disorders, not all cases can be explained this way. Dr. Gallagher provides several fascinating case studies and advocates for a balanced approach to the subject of possession that respects both scientific skepticism and the experiences of those who believe in the demonic phenomena.

29. Mark 8:33; Matthew 16:23 (KJV).

30. Job 1–2.

31. Luke 10:19 (NLT).

32. Isaiah 54:17.

33. Ephesians 6:12.

34. Acts 19:13 (NLT).

35. Acts 19:15–16 (NLT).

36. Revelation 2:20–24 (NASB).

Chapter 9

1. Ephesians 2:2 (NLT).

2. Genesis 6:2–8.

3. 2 Corinthians 2:11.

4. John 6:35.

5. 2 Corinthians 4:4.

6. John 10:10.

7. John 8:34.

8. 1 Thessalonians 5:23.

9. Ephesians 2:1.

10. 2 Corinthians 4:3–4.

11. Psalm 14:1.

12. Proverbs 6:16–19; 1 John 2:15.

13. John 1:12 (NLT).

14. Hebrews 12:6 (NLT).

15. Psalm 37:4.

16. Hebrews 4:12.

17. 2 Corinthians 4:4 (NLT).

18. For an in-depth and scholarly analysis of the Bible, I highly recommend the book *Evidence that Demands a Verdict*, written by Josh McDowell, a former skeptic who initially set out to prove the Bible untrue only to come to an altogether different conclusion.

19. Genesis 2:16–17 (NLT).

20. Genesis 3:1 (NLT).

21. Genesis 3:1–6 (NLT).

22. Richard Swenson, *Margin: Restoring Emotional, Physical, Financial, and Time Reserves to Overloaded Lives* (Tyndale House, 2014).

23. Revelation 7:9.

24. 1 Corinthians 8:1; Proverbs 1:7.

25. Varun Warrier et al., "Elevated Rates of Autism, Other Neurodevelopmental and Psychiatric Diagnoses, and Autistic Traits in Transgender and Gender-Diverse Individuals," *Nature Communications* 11, no. 1 (August 2020), 3959, https://www.nature.com/articles/s41467-020-17794-1.

26. Hebrews 2:15.

27. John 8:34; Romans 6:23.

28. 1 Corinthians 15:19 (AMP).

29. John 3:16.

30. *The Hunger Games*, directed by Gary Ross (Lionsgate, 2012).

31. 1 Corinthians 15:26.

Chapter 10

1. Genesis 50:20.

2. Exodus 1:8 (KJV).

3. 1 Peter 2:9.

4. Colossians 1:13.

5. John 6:44; John 12:32; Ezekiel 34:11; Proverbs 8:17.

6. Galatians 4:7.

7. 2 Corinthians 5:18–21.

8. Matthew 28:18–20.

9. United States v. Wilson. 32 U.S. 150 (1833).

10. Hebrews 2:8 (NKJV).

11. Ezekiel 28:16–17; Isaiah 14:12; Revelation 12:7–9.

12. Revelation 12:12.

13. Mark 12:30–31 (NLT); Deuteronomy 6:5; Leviticus 19:18; Matthew 22:37–39; Luke 10:27.

14. James 1:25 (Berean Standard Bible).

15. Viktor E. Frankl, *The Doctor and the Soul: From Psychotherapy to Logotherapy* (Vintage, 1986), 53–54.

16. 2 Timothy 2:4.

17. 1 Peter 1:7.

18. 2 Timothy 2:21 (NLT).

19. 2 Corinthians 12:7 (NLT).

20. 2 Corinthians 12:7–8 (NLT).

21. Hebrews 11:25 (CSB).

22. Romans 8:28.

23. Jeremiah 29:11; Romans 8:28.

24. Luke 9:62.

25. James 4:4 (NLT).

26. John 14:27 (NLT).

27. 1 John 2:17.

28. Matthew 12:30; Luke 11:23 (ESV).

29. 1 Corinthians 10:12 (AMP).

30. Revelation 12:10.

31. Hebrews 7:25 (NLT).

32. Romans 8:1–2 (NLT).

33. Revelation 19:7–9.

34. John 10:11, 14.

35. Ephesians 4:11.

36. John 10:1.

37. Matthew 7:16–20.

38. Jude 1:4.

39. 1 Timothy 4:1.

40. 2 Corinthians 11:4.

41. Matthew 24:5 (KJV).

42. Lewis, *Mere Christianity*, 52.

43. 2 Thessalonians 2:9.

44. Acts 8:9–11; Exodus 7, 8.

45. 1 John 4:1–3.

46. 1 Corinthians 2:14.

47. Mark 16:15 (NKJV).

48. 2 Corinthians 4:4; Isaiah 8:14–15; Romans 9:33; 1 Peter 2:8.

49. 2 Timothy 4:2–4 (NASB).

50. Romans 8:37 (KJV).

51. Romans 8:37; Joshua 1:9.

Chapter 11

1. Hebrews 4:12.

2. Matthew 23:26 (NLT).

3. Adrian Rogers, "Guard Your Heart," Oneplace, https://www.oneplace.com/ministries/love-worth-finding/read/articles/guard-your-heart-17739.html.

4. Proverbs 4:23 (NLT); 23:7 (AMPC).

5. John 7:24; 1 Samuel 16:7; Jeremiah 17:10.

6. Ephesians 4:18; Mark 7:21.

7. Psalm 51:10; Ezekiel 36:26; Romans 12:2; Ephesians 4:23.

8. Lewis, *Mere Christianity*, 3–31.

9. Lewis, *Mere Christianity*.

10. Philippians 2:13.

11. Jeremiah 17:9 (NLT).

12. 1 Corinthians 2:14–16.

13. 1 Peter 5:8; Proverbs 4:23; Luke 12:35–40; Mark 14:38; 1 Thessalonians 5:6.

14. 2 Corinthians 10:3–5.

15. Matthew 7:1–5 (KJV).

16. Revelation 2:20–22.

17. Deuteronomy 18:10–12a (NIV).

18. 1 Timothy 4:1.

19. 2 Corinthians 10:4.

20. Philippians 4:8 (NLT).

21. 2 Corinthians 10:5 (KJV).

22. Romans 12:2 (NLT).

23. Ephesians 4:21–23 (NLT).

24. John Wesley, *Renew My Heart* (Barbour Publishing, 2011), 193.

25. 1 Peter 1:13–14; Romans 1:18.

26. Philippians 4:7.

27. John Bunyan, *The Holy War* (Whittaker House, 2001).

28. Galatians 5:22–23.

29. Romans 8:1 (NLT).

30. 1 John 2:16 (NLT).

31. Romans 8:16.

32. 2 Timothy 1:7.

33. Romans 1:28–32; 8:6–8.

34. 1 Peter 5:8; 4:7; 1:13; Titus 2:12; Ephesians 5:18; 2 Timothy 4:5; 1 Thessalonians 5:8.

35. Mark 5:15; Luke 8:35; 15:17; 1 Corinthians 15:34.

36. Hebrews 4:12.

Chapter 12

1. Jean Twenge et al., "Age, Period, and Cohort Trends in Mood Disorder Indicators and Suicide-Related Outcomes in a Nationally Representative Dataset, 2005–2017," *Journal of Abnormal Psychology* 128, no. 3 (April 2019), 185–99.

2. Eileen Crimmins et al., "Changing Disease Prevalence, Incidence, and Mortality Among Older Cohorts: The Health and Retirement Study," *The Journals of Gerontology: Series A* 75, issue supplement 1 (December 2019), S21–S26, https://doi.org/10.1093/gerona/glz075.

3. George Engel, "The Biopsychosocial Model and the Education of Health Professionals," *Annals of the New York Academy of Science* 310, no. 1 (June 1978), 169–81, https://doi.org/10.1111/j.1749-6632.1978.tb22070.x.

4. Frankl, *The Doctor and the Soul*, xxiv.

5. Denise McKee and John Chappel, "Spirituality and Medical Practice," *Journal of Family Practice* 35, no. 2 (August 1992), 201–5, http://cdn.mdedge.com/files/s3fs-public/jfp-archived-issues/1992-volume_34/JFP_1992-08_v35_i2_spirituality-and-medical-practice.pdf.

6. Harold Koenig, *Spirituality and Health Research: Methods, Measurements, Statistics, and Resources* (Templeton Foundation Press, 2012), 27.

7. Koenig, *Spirituality and Health Research*, 14.

8. Megan Best, Phyllis Butow, and Ian Olver, "Doctors Discussing Religion and Spirituality: A Systematic Literature Review," *Palliative Medicine* 30, no. 4 (April 2016), 327–37, https://doi.org/10.1177/0269216315600912.

9. Best, Butow, and Olver, "Doctors Discussing Religion."

10. Lusine Poghosyan et al., "Mental Health Delivery in Primary Care: The Perspectives of Primary Care Providers," *Archives of Psychiatric Nursing* 33, no. 5 (October 2019), 63–67, https://doi.org/10.1016/j.apnu.2019.08.001.

11. "Constitution," World Health Organization, https://www.who.int/about/governance/constitution.

12. 2 Corinthians 10:4.

13. *Alcoholics Anonymous: The Story of How Many Thousands of Men and Women Have Recovered from Alcoholism*, 4th ed. (Alcoholics Anonymous World Services, Inc., 2001), 64.

14. John Kelly, Keith Humphreys, and Marica Ferri, "Alcoholics Anonymous and Other 12-Step Programs for Alcohol Use Disorder," *Cochrane Database of Systemic Reviews*, no. 3 (March 2020), https://doi.org/10.1002/14651858. CD012880.pub2.

15. While the 12 Steps of Ruachiatry in this book were inspired by the Twelve Steps of Alcoholics Anonymous, they are not really an adaptation. Rather, they were created specifically for this publication, and should not be construed otherwise. A.A. is a program concerned only with recovery from alcoholism and is not in any way affiliated with nor does it endorse this publication. If you need help with a drinking problem, want to know more about A.A., or want to find A.A. near you, resources are provided at: www.aa.org.

Chapter 13

1. Elisabeth Kübler-Ross and David Kessler, *On Grief and Grieving* (Simon & Schuster, 2014).

2. Frankl, *The Doctor and the Soul*, 44.

3. Ecclesiastes 5:18–19 (NLT).

4. Ephesians 6:10–13 (AMP).

5. *Rocky II*, directed by Sylvester Stallone (United Artists, 1979).

6. David Martyn Lloyd-Jones, *The Christian Soldier* (Baker Books, 1977), 17–18.

7. Psalm 145:14 (NLT).

8. 2 Chronicles 16:12 (NLT).

9. B. Leurent et al., "Spiritual and Religious Beliefs as Risk Factors for the Onset of Major Depression: An International Cohort Study," *Psychological Medicine* 43, no. 10 (October 2018), 2109–20, https://doi.org/10.1017/S0033291712003066.

10. Michael King et al., "Religion, Spirituality and Mental Health: Results from a National Study of English Households," *The British Journal of Psychiatry* 202, no. 1 (January 2013), 68–73, https://doi.org/10.1192/bjp.bp.112.112003.

11. Matthew 7:7; Hebrews 11:6; Psalm 119:2; Deuteronomy 4:29; Acts 17:27; Proverbs 8:17; Jeremiah 29:13.

12. Isaiah 55:8–9.

13. Exodus 15:26.

14. This title and concept appear throughout biblical literature to affirm faith in God's power to heal both physical and spiritual ailments, but it is first mentioned in Exodus 15:26.

15. 1 John 2:16 (NKJV).

16. Frankl, *The Doctor and the Soul*, 40.

17. 1 John 2:16.

18. 1 John 2:16.

19. Exodus 20:3 (KJV).

20. Matthew 22:36–40; Mark 10:28–31; Luke 10:27.

21. Matthew 16:24.

22. Luke 22:42 (NLT).

23. John 6:38.

24. Matthew 6:10.

25. Isaiah 14:13–14 (NKJV).

26. Psalm 44:21.

27. Ephesians 6:15.

28. Matthew 16:18.

29. Romans 8:31 (NKJV).

30. Deuteronomy 31:6; Hebrews 13:5; 1 Kings 8:57; Genesis 28:15.

31. Psalm 23:4.

32. John 17:15.

33. 2 Corinthians 12:7 (NLT).

34. 2 Corinthians 12:7–10 (NLT).

35. Philippians 4:7.

36. Romans 8:28 (Berean Standard Bible).

37. Wesley, *Renew My Heart*, 100.

38. James 2:17.

39. Matthew 7:21 (NLT).

40. 2 Corinthians 4:17.

Chapter 14

1. 2 Corinthians 10:1 (NIV).

2. Proverbs 28:1.

3. This quote is commonly attributed to Epictetus, but there is no direct record of this exact wording in his surviving works. Instead, it likely paraphrases a central idea from his teachings on emotional self-control, particularly as found in *The Enchiridion* (or Manual), which emphasizes the importance of not letting external circumstances or people control one's emotions.

4. Wesley, *Renew My Heart*, 208.

5. Isaiah 53:7–11; Mark 15:2–5; John 19:9–11; Matthew 27:11–14; Luke 23:8–16.

6. Matthew 21:12–13; Mark 11:15–17; Luke 19:45–47; John 2:15–17.

7. Hebrews 12:15.

8. Ephesians 4:31–32 (NIV).

9. Ecclesiastes 7:9 (NLT).

10. Proverbs 4:23 (NLT).

11. Matthew 5:21–26.

12. 1 Peter 2:23 (NLT).

13. Romans 12:19 (AMP).

14. Proverbs 20:22 (NLT).

15. Colossians 3:13; Ephesians 4:32; Isaiah 1:18; Mark 11:25; Matthew 6:14.

16. Matthew 18:32–35 (NLT).

17. 1 Corinthians 13:4–5.

18. Proverbs 17:9 (NLT).

19. 1 John 1:9.

20. Matthew 5:23–24 (NIV).

21. 1 Samuel 15:22.

22. Lucas S. LaFreniere and Michelle G. Newman, "Exposing Worry's Deceit: Percentage of Untrue Worries in Generalized Anxiety Disorder Treatment," *Behavior Therapy* 51, no. 3 (May 2020), 413–23, https://doi.org/10.1016/j.beth.2019.07.003.

23. This quote is widely attributed to Emerson, but the phrase does not appear in his published works or collected writings.

24. I give credit here to the late pastor of First Baptist Church of Atlanta and former president of the Southern Baptist Convention, Dr. Charles Stanley, who frequently made this statement in his sermons.

25. Hebrews 11:6.

26. 2 Corinthians 5:7 (KJV).

27. Psalm 28:7; Genesis 15:1; Psalm 3:3.

28. Hebrews 2:15 (NLT).

29. John 8:36.

30. 2 Corinthians 10:4.

31. 2 Timothy 1:7 (NKJV).

32. Psalm 46:1–2.

33. 1 Peter 5:7 (NIV).

34. 1 Peter 5:8.

35. Ephesians 5:18.

36. Ephesians 4:27.

37. James 4:7.

38. Matthew 12:43–45; Luke 11:24–26.

39. Philippians 4:8 (GNT).

40. Romans 12:2.

Chapter 15

1. Romans 3:11.

2. Deuteronomy 31:6.

3. Isaiah 55:11; 2 Timothy 3:16–17; Psalm 85:8; Jeremiah 33:3; John 10:27.

4. 2 Timothy 2:3.

5. 2 Timothy 3:15.

6. Ecclesiastes 1:17; 12:13 (NLT).

7. Psalm 111:10; Proverbs 9:10.

8. 1 John 2:17; 1 Corinthians 7:31; Matthew 24:35; Luke21:33; Psalm 119:89; Isaiah 40:8.

9. Wikipedia, s.v. "Occult," last modified April 14, 2025, https://en.wikipedia.org/wiki/Occult#Notes.

10. Deuteronomy 18:9–12; Isaiah 8:19; 44:25; Jeremiah 27:9; 2 Kings 21:6; 23:24.

11. Ian Barbour, *When Science meets Religion: Enemies, Strangers, or Partners?* (Harper Collins, 2020).

12. Lloyd-Jones, *The Christian Soldier*, 333.

13. Matthew 4:4; Luke 4:4.

14. Ephesians 6:17.

15. Hebrews 4:11 (NLT).

16. Matthew 3:16–17; Mark 1:9–11; Luke 3:21–22.

17. Matthew 4:1–11; Luke 4:1–13.

18. Hebrews 4:15 (NIV).

19. 1 Peter 5:8.

20. Luke 4:13 (AMP).

21. John 17:17 (AMPC).

22. James 4:4.

23. Romans 12:2 (NLT).

24. Matthew 13:43.

25. Romans 8:18 (NKJV).

26. Colossians 2:11 (NLT).

27. Proverbs 23:7.

28. Romans 8:6; Romans 6:18–22.

29. 2 Timothy 3:16 (NLT).

30. Jeremiah 15:16; Matthew 4:4.

31. Hebrews 4:16.

32. Mark 1:35.

33. Matthew 6:7 (AMP and ESV).

34. Luke 18:1.

35. Ephesians 6:18 (NIV).

36. 1 Thessalonians 5:16; Ephesians 6:18.

37. Psalm 46:1.

38. Hebrews 1:3.

39. Hebrews 4:16 (NLT).

40. Psalm 38:3; 17–18.

41. Psalm 32:3–4.

42. 1 John 1:9 (NET).

43. Deuteronomy 10:14; 1 Chronicles 29:14; Romans 11:36; James 1:17.

44. Matthew 7:7; Luke 11:9; Psalm 37:4; 1 John 5:14–15.

45. Philippians 4:6 (AMPC).

46. 1 Corinthians 12:20–27.

47. Hebrews 10:25.

48. James 5:16 (NLT).

49. Ephesians 6:18.

50. Psalm 37:7.

51. Isaiah 40:31.

52. 1 Kings 19:12; Ecclesiastes 5:2.

53. 2 Corinthians 3:3; Jeremiah 31:33; Hebrews 8:10.

54. Joshua 1:8; Psalm 1:2.

55. Michael Balboni et al., "Nurse and Physician Barriers to Spiritual Care Provision at the End of Life," *Journal of Pain and Symptom Management* 48, no. 3 (September 2014), 400–410, https://doi.org/10.1016/j.jpainsymman.2013.09.020; Tracy Balboni et al., "Religiousness and Spiritual Support Among Advanced Cancer Patients and Associations with End-Of-Life Treatment Preferences and Quality Of Life," *Journal of Clinical Oncology* 25, no. 5 (February 2007), 555–60, https://doi.org/10.1200/JCO.2006.07.9046.

56. Matthew 15:14 (KJV).

57. Proverbs 15:8 (NLT).

Epilogue

1. Isaiah 55:3 (NLT).

2. Numbers 21:5–7.

3. John 3:14–15 (NLT).

4. Galatians 3:13.

5. 2 Corinthians 5:21 (NIV).

6. John 5:1–18.

7. John 16:33.

8. John 16:20.

9. 2 Corinthians 4:17.

10. John 16:21–22.

11. 2 Corinthians 4:18.

12. Isaiah 30:20–21 (NLT).

13. Psalms 119:71 (NLT).

14. Michael Heiser, *The Unseen Realm: Recovering the Supernatural Worldview of the Bible* (Lexham Press, 2015), 158, 263, 344, 353, 383. This concept was first developed by Princeton theologian Geerhardus Vos in the early twentieth century.

15. Hebrews 2:8 (NKJV).

16. John 11:1–44 (NLT).

17. Hebrews 4:15 (NIV).

18. Romans 5:2b–6 (NLT).

19. 2 Corinthians 5:18 (NLT).

For permission to reproduce copyrighted material, grateful acknowledgment is made to the following.

ABOUT THE AUTHOR

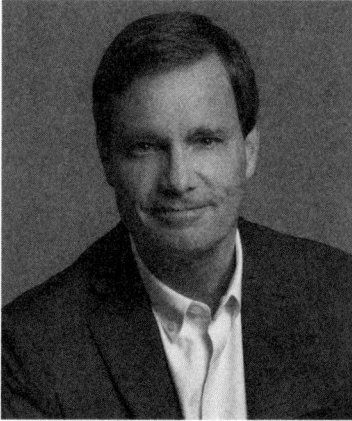

Thomas W. McCormack, MD, is a psychiatrist, educator, and thought leader in the integration of spirituality and medicine. Dr. McCormack earned his medical degree from Emory University School of Medicine, completed his residency and two fellowships at Duke University, and has been awarded board certifications in general psychiatry, child and adolescent psychiatry, and forensic psychiatry.

Dr. McCormack has built a thriving multidisciplinary practice in Athens, Georgia, specializing in complex and treatment-resistant psychiatric cases. He has also served as a clinical assistant professor at Emory University and is currently at the UGA School of Medicine.

Beyond his clinical and legal expertise, he is actively involved in civic activities, holding leadership positions in his church and contributing to nonprofit organizations that support mental health and youth services.

Dr. McCormack lives in Athens, Georgia, with his wife, Michelle, and they have three beloved adult children.

Visit www.Ruachiatry.org and www.Hidden-Medicine.com to learn more.